# CAREGIVER RESOURCES:

## From Independence to a Memory Care Unit

*Laura Town, Karen Kassel,*
*and Amanda Boyle*

Silver Hills Press
Zionsville, IN 46077

ISBN: 978-1-943414-01-7

**Production Credits:**
**Authors:** Laura Town, Karen Kassel, and Amanda Boyle
**Publisher:** Silver Hills Press
**Photos:** All images used under license from Shutterstock.com

**Social Media Connections:**
**Laura Town**
Twitter: @laurawtown
LinkedIn: https://www.linkedin.com/in/lauratown
GooglePlus: https://plus.google.com/u/0/117415714202281042310/posts
Pinterest: https://www.pinterest.com/laurat0428

**Karen Kassel**
Twitter: @KarenKassel1
LinkedIn: www.linkedin.com/pub/karen-kassel/62/2b/915/

**Amanda Boyle**
Twitter: @AmandaLBoyle
LinkedIn: www.linkedin.com/pub/amanda-boyle/45/406/191

# TABLE OF CONTENTS

# CAREGIVER RESOURCES: FROM INDEPENDENCE TO A MEMORY CARE UNIT

Alzheimer's disease is a progressive condition, worsening in terms of physical symptoms and cognitive decline as the disease moves into the later stages. In the early stages of the disease, when your loved is first diagnosed, they will likely continue daily activities without many changes to their routine or lifestyle. However, as the condition worsens, you will gradually need to make changes to ensure the safety and overall well-being of your loved one. These changes may be minor home repairs and precautions, but they could also include relocation and dedicated medical assistance. As you make these changes, you will find that one painful aspect of caring for a loved one with Alzheimer's disease is trying to balance their psychological need for independence with their physical safety. Living arrangements impact both independence and safety and should be discussed as early as possible so that your loved one can make their preferences known.

On average, individuals with Alzheimer's disease live ten years past their diagnosis. In those ten years, they will likely change living arrangements several times as the disease progresses. None of these changes are easy, and each one has its own unique challenges. In the early stages of the disease, your loved one can likely stay at home, but as the symptoms worsen, other options will need to be considered. For example, in my (Laura's) situation, Dad lived at home independently for a short period of time, then he lived at home with us checking on him twice a day, then he had 24-hour at-home care, then he moved into an assisted living facility, and then he went into a nursing home. Each situation had its own financial and emotional stressors for me, my dad, and my family, and each required careful consideration about Dad's autonomy and well-being.

Finding the living arrangement that works best for your loved one, as well as you and your family, is very important, and what is best will likely change as the disease progresses. Every situation is different, so while living with a caregiver might be the perfect option for one family, an assisted living facility or long-term care facility could be the best solution for another family. Before making these decisions, you must know the facts concerning each type of facility, understand the considerations involved in choosing the right facility, and recognize the safety concerns associated with each option. Alzheimer's disease has become much more prevalent in recent years. Therefore, many care providers and housing facilities have dedicated staff who are trained to work with individuals who have this disease. However, this is not always the case, so it is important to research the background and training requirements of any facility you and your loved one are considering.

# Staying at Home

Most of us would prefer to live in our homes unaided until our death. Although it is unlikely that your loved one with Alzheimer's disease will be able to do this, they will probably choose to stay at home as long they can. In the beginning, this will not involve a lot of planning or changes around the house, but as the disease progresses, changes must be made for both convenience and safety. Additional help may be needed for daily cleaning tasks, laundry, maintenance, or companionship. When working with your loved one to make changes around the house or to their daily routine, try to ensure that these changes will not negatively impact their sense of independence. This can be difficult to balance, but preserving as much of their independence as possible will make a huge difference to your loved one.

## Preserving Independence

Helping your loved one preserve their independence is important for someone in the early stages of Alzheimer's disease. This is important not only because your loved one will want as much independence as possible, but also because it can help increase and preserve your loved one's mental acuity. You might feel compelled to take control of everything the moment your loved one is diagnosed with Alzheimer's disease because you think doing so will help relieve some of their burden or stress. In fact, the exact opposite is likely to happen. Upon being diagnosed with Alzheimer's disease, your loved one will begin to realize that soon it will be impossible to do many of the things they once enjoyed. This realization will turn any loss of independence, no matter how small, into a sign of what is to come in the future. The following checklist discusses tips for helping your loved one maintain independence while they still live at home.

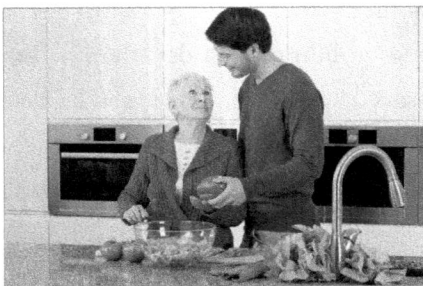

2

## Checklist: Helping preserve independence while living at home

☐ Avoid taking control. In the early stages of Alzheimer's disease, your loved one can still do many things on their own, so only offer help when needed.

☐ Help your loved one set up automatic bill payments for their monthly bills.

☐ For bills that cannot be set up through bill pay (snow removal, local newspaper delivery, landscaping, etc.), suggest that your loved one create a calendar with dates for when these payments need to be made. Once each check is delivered, your loved one can cross the corresponding payment off the calendar.

☐ Help your loved one set up daily routines to make the management of daily tasks easier and less stressful. Be observant about tasks that are going undone in your loved one's home (e.g., cleaning, laundry, grocery shopping) and offer to help. Your loved one may be resistant to ask for help with everyday tasks, but if you offer, they may be less hesitant to accept.

☐ Post clear instructions for common appliances such as the washer, dryer, stove, oven, dishwasher, phone, TV, shower, and toilet. This will help your loved one know how to use these appliances if they get confused or can't remember.

☐ If your loved one has trouble with incontinence, place incontinence pads close to the toilet for your loved one to use.

☐ If your loved one used to enjoy going for walks (or other similar activities) but has stopped due to a fear of getting confused or lost, offer to go for a walk with them on a set day or two each week.

☐ If your loved one has a pet, post reminders to feed the pet, take it outside to use the bathroom, or complete other needed pet care chores.

☐ Buy an electric tea kettle so that your loved one can make tea or instant coffee without having to worry about forgetting the stove is on. Make sure you purchase a device with an automatic shut-off feature.

☐ Stock the refrigerator and pantry with easy-to-make foods, such as sandwich materials or meals that can be made in the microwave. If your loved one has experienced problems using the microwave, consider posting directions for microwave use nearby.

- [ ] If your loved one enjoys cooking, offer to help them cook a few meals each week, but make sure not to take over. Allow your loved one to do as much of the preparation as possible, only lending support when necessary.

- [ ] If your loved one is used to doing the grocery shopping, help them create a grocery list so the trip is easier.

- [ ] If becoming confused at the grocery store is a concern, offer to go with your loved one. Be there for support and companionship, but do not interfere unless they need or ask for your help. Alternately, you could help your loved one create an online shopping list and have the groceries delivered to their home.

## Meals on Wheels

If your loved one can no longer cook and you are not able to help, arrange with Meals on Wheels to deliver hot meals to your loved one. Meals on Wheels America is a senior nutrition program that works to ensure no elder adult goes without food. Approximately one million meals per day are provided by Meals on Wheels in the United States, with options to deliver either breakfast, lunch, or dinner. These meals are served at senior centers or can be delivered straight to a person's home. The checklist below discusses some of the aspects of this program.

### *Checklist: Basics about the Meals on Wheels program*

- [ ] The individual receiving meals must be homebound (not able to leave the home, or has difficultly leaving the home) and at least 60 years old. Those under age 60 can also receive meals if they have a disability or meet income requirements. Requirements differ by state and program, so check with your local organization to see if your loved one qualifies.

- [ ] Prices per meal are generally set on a sliding scale but can be anywhere from free to $8 a meal. Some areas offer meal packages where you can pay for meals by the week.

- [ ] Meals on Wheels programs employ nutritionists, so meals are healthy and well balanced. All meals satisfy one-third of an individual's daily recommended nutrition and include grains, protein, and vegetables; milk, bread, and dessert are also often provided.

- [ ] You can sign a loved one up to have meals delivered to their house; individuals do not have to sign themselves up for the program. You will need to fill out an application (or answer questions over the phone) regarding any dietary restrictions your loved one has. Once signed up, meal delivery can generally start within a day or two

- [ ] Meals are generally only served on weekdays (Monday through Friday), but frozen meals can be provided for the weekends if needed.

- [ ] For individuals who have meals delivered weekly, nonperishable food items are delivered in advance of very bad weather. This way, if a volunteer cannot make it to your loved one's home because of the weather, food is still available. In some states (Pennsylvania, Maryland, Washington, and others), Meals on Wheels programs offer grocery shopping services to homebound seniors. Sometimes $5–$10 is charged for this service in addition to the cost of groceries.

- [ ] Some programs will also provide pet food at a discounted rate once a month for seniors who have pets living with them.

- [ ] Meals on Wheels has programs across the country in both rural and urban areas. You can use the following website to find a provider near you: http://www.mealsonwheelsamerica.org. Additional contact information for this program can be found in the Resources section at the end of the book.

## Home Modifications for Independence

In order for your loved one to safely stay in their home, you may need to make several modifications. These changes are meant to increase your loved one's independence and overall well-being and to promote their safety. Changes made to reduce disorientation and promote independence are among the simpler, less expensive changes that will be needed. The following checklist details some of these changes.

### Checklist: Home modifications to reduce confusion

- [ ] Have an accurate clock in every room so your loved one can be aware of the passing of time and use it to orient their mind to the time of day.

- [ ] Hang a calendar with large numbers in the room in which your loved one spends the most time. You or your loved one can cross days off as they pass, and you can also add appointments to the calendar to help your loved one remember them.

- [ ] Avoid rearranging rooms in the house unless the change is needed for safety reasons.

- [ ] Purchase a digital voice reminder device for the door your loved one uses to exit the house. These reminders will sound when the door opens; a voice recording will instruct your loved one to turn off the lights and remember the house keys, or it will play whatever messages you program into the device.

- [ ] Hang signs with the room name on or next to the door for common rooms, such as the bedroom, bathroom, and kitchen. This will help your loved one find the needed room if they get disoriented. If needed, add an explanation of the purpose of the room.

- [ ] Close doors and post "keep out" signs for rooms that your loved one does not need to use.

- [ ] Get rid of excess or unneeded clothing to decrease choices, which will help eliminate some stress.

- [ ] Remove all excess clutter from the house.

- [ ] Ensure that stairways are well lit; this could include adding light switches at the top and bottom of each stairwell.

- [ ] Add reflective and/or colorful tape to the edge of stairs to increase visibility.

- [ ] Install extra lighting in all rooms.

## Promoting Safety

Unlike most independence-related modifications, changes to the house for safety reasons can be expensive, but they are necessary and can prevent greater expenses later on. Some safety-related modifications are made to prevent falling and tripping. Others include locking up medications and hazardous products such as cleaning solutions and guns. Still others aim to reduce the likelihood of wandering or automobile accidents. Additional measures address oft-overlooked but equally important issues, such as disaster safety and suicide prevention.

## Fall Safety

Preventing falls should be a high priority for you and your loved one. Older adults, even those without cognitive impairment, are at high risk of falling, which may result in fractured bones or other injuries. Individuals with Alzheimer's disease are at an even higher risk of falling than other older adults, because they may not process the presence of obstacles, they have a reduced sense of balance, and they may make poor decisions about climbing and reaching.

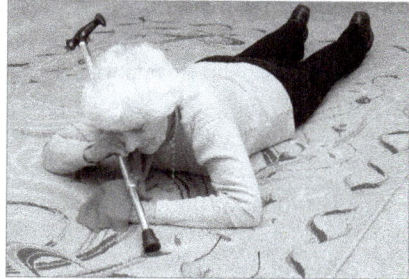

The thought of Dad falling was one of the many nightmares I had as a caregiver. For me, the key to preventing Dad from falling was making sure that he had good, sturdy shoes on at all times and keeping every room free of clutter. The checklists below provide some simple changes you can make to help reduce the risk of falling.

### Checklist: Outdoor modifications

- ☐ Keep walkways clear of debris.
- ☐ Fix loose or uneven steps.
- ☐ Add a railing next to walkways and stairs.
- ☐ Install a ramp to the front and back doors.

### Checklist: Indoor modifications

**Kitchen:**

- ☐ Keep commonly used dishes and utensils within easy reach to prevent climbing and reaching.
- ☐ If you need to polish the floor, use a nonslip cleaner. You may need to test several cleaners to determine which one works best for your flooring. Encourage your loved one to stay out of the kitchen when the floor is wet.
- ☐ Clean up spills immediately.

**Bathroom:**

☐ Remove all rugs that may slip; secure remaining rugs or use nonskid mats. Rugs can be secured using nonslip rubber rug pads, double-sided tape, or glue. Different floor types require different methods of securing a rug, and different rugs may need different methods as well, depending on the rug backing.

☐ Add nonslip decals to the bottom of the shower or tub.

☐ Install a faucet cover in the bathtub to reduce injury if your loved one falls.

☐ Install grab bars in the shower and next to the toilet.

☐ Install a raised toilet seat.

☐ Install an anchored shower bench and a hand-held sprayer.

☐ Install a walk-in shower or tub so your loved one doesn't have to climb over the side of the tub.

**Living spaces:**

☐ Keep all walking areas free from clutter.

☐ Remove or secure rugs that may cause tripping.

☐ Make sure all electrical cords are secured to the floor and out of walking paths.

☐ Remove low furniture that may present a tripping hazard. Low furniture is furniture that is below knee-level, such as a coffee table.

☐ Encourage the use of assistive devices when walking; ensure that walking paths are wide enough to accommodate use of assistive devices.

☐ Provide your loved one with good, sturdy shoes that have rubber soles to prevent slipping. Make sure they wear the shoes at all times except when sleeping. Shoes with Velcro straps are preferred because some individuals with Alzheimer's disease may forget how to tie their shoes, leaving laces loose; or they may remove shoelaces, increasing the chances of the shoes falling off. This then presents another tripping hazard.

☐ Provide adequate lighting of all hallways and living spaces, especially at night. Use nightlights or motion-sensing lights as necessary. Because individuals with

Alzheimer's disease have visual difficulties, inadequate lighting can cause confusion and misperceptions.

☐ Install handrails in all stairways; handrails should extend beyond the first and last steps.

☐ Install safety gates at the top and bottom of stairways. Be sure to install a gate that works best with your loved one's stairs and not one that tips easily.

☐ Add nonskid, colored strips to each stair. This helps define the stairs for individuals who have difficulty with depth perception due to similar colors.

☐ Be aware that pets can become tripping hazards, especially if they are a similar color as the carpet. If necessary, you may need to find these pets a new home.

**Bedroom:**

☐ Place clothing and shoes in easy-to-reach locations.

☐ Install side rails on the bed or use a hospital bed.

☐ Anticipate needs that might require your loved one to walk at night; make sure they have gone to the bathroom and are not hungry or thirsty before bedtime.

It may be beneficial to enroll your loved one in an emergency alert system such as Lifeline. With most emergency alert systems, your loved one will wear a pendant with a button they can push to call for help. Extra emergency alert buttons can be mounted near the floor in common areas or in areas that an individual may land in when they fall, such as the bottom of the stairway. Lifeline also has an auto-alert option that calls for help if it detects a fall and your loved one is unable to push the button. You can order a Lifeline system online at www.lifelinesys.com or call at 1-844-448-1403. Other emergency alert companies are listed in the Resources section at the end of this book.

## Hazard Safety

Individuals with Alzheimer's disease often have impaired perception and judgment. Therefore, they may not realize that something is dangerous. For example, they may touch a hot stove, eat a poisonous plant, or drink a clear liquid that happens to be bleach. They may also struggle with basic activities that have been routine for them in the past, giving rise to unexpected dangers. For example, my dad tried to make a frozen pizza, which he was an expert at, having been a bachelor for some time. One day he just turned on the burners and placed the cardboard box with the pizza on top. We were fortunate that he didn't burn himself or burn the house down. From that moment on, I made sure that his fridge was stocked with sandwich makings, and we had Meals on Wheels bring him warm meals.

When caring for someone with Alzheimer's disease, you must learn to never underestimate a potential hazard. As a caregiver, removing hazardous substances or keeping them in a locked cabinet could save your loved one from potential injury or death. Hazard safety tips for individuals with Alzheimer's disease are included in the checklists below.

### Checklist: Personal safety

- ☐ Label or color-code hot (red) and cold (blue) water faucets or install a faucet with only one handle that controls both hot and cold water.

- ☐ Set the hot water heater to 120 °F to avoid scalding. If your loved one's water heater temperature control is not reliable, consider replacing the water heater with a more reliable unit.

- ☐ Place red tape around heating sources to deter your loved one from touching them when hot.

- ☐ Remove or lock up sharp objects such as knives, razors, and scissors.

- ☐ Only allow your loved one to use an electric razor for shaving to prevent cuts.

- ☐ Consider disabling the garbage disposal, as individuals with Alzheimer's disease may stick their hand or other items into the disposal when it is running.

- ☐ Put away small appliances such as toasters and blenders when not in use.

- ☐ Use appliances that have an automatic shut-off feature.

- ☐ Keep appliances away from water sources, including bathroom appliances such as hair dryers and electric razors.

- ☐ Keep the refrigerator clear of spoiled foods, because your loved one may not be able to smell that the food is bad.

- ☐ Remove small items that may be easily swallowed; lock the "junk" drawer that may contain these items.

- ☐ Remove plastic fruit and magnets that may be mistaken for food and eaten.

- ☐ Replace breakable glass with plastic. This applies to glass tables, glass shower doors, drinking glasses, and ceramic plates.

- ☐ Mark windows and glass doors with decals to help your loved one see the panes.

- ☐ Make sure that carbon monoxide detectors are installed and working properly; change batteries at least once a year. Carbon monoxide detectors should be placed near sleeping areas and main living areas but not close to a furnace unit.

- ☐ Remove fish tanks or keep them out of reach, because they pose an electrocution hazard.

- ☐ Remove poisonous plants from the home.

- ☐ Store power tools in a locked area to which your loved one doesn't have a key.

- ☐ Disable automatic locks so your loved one does not get locked out accidentally.

- ☐ Hide an extra house key outside in case your loved one locks everyone out.

- ☐ Install coverings or doors to conceal rooms that may pose a hazard to your loved one.

- ☐ Have a first aid kit readily available.

- ☐ Keep emergency contact numbers in easy reach of all phones. Program phones with speed dial for caregivers and emergency personnel, and make a list of the numbers in large font (e.g., 1 = daughter, 2 = police, etc.) and place it next to the phone. If desired, you could use photos to accompany the list. Leave clear, simple directions next to the phone for your loved one to follow.

## Checklist: Fire safety

- ☐ Make sure that smoke detectors are installed to code and working; change batteries at least once a year.

- ☐ Keep fire extinguishers in easily accessible locations; you should have one in every room if possible.

- ☐ Use child safety covers for all outlets when not in use.

☐ Keep matches and lighters locked up or out of reach.

☐ Consider disabling the stove, oven, and microwave when not in use. For example, remove the knobs on the stove or install a hidden circuit breaker.

☐ If you decide to keep the microwave or stove functional, place clear, simple directions next to it for your loved one to follow. Make sure papers stay clear of the heating elements.

☐ Remove space heaters and hot plates; do not let your loved one control settings for electric blankets or heating pads.

☐ Remove the fuel source for all grills when not in use.

☐ Supervise or restrict smoking. If your loved one must smoke, make sure someone is with them at all times. Cigarettes can be a fire hazard if left on flammable material.

☐ Supervise the use of the fireplace and candles; always extinguish the fire when leaving your loved one alone in a room with an open flame.

## Checklist: Chemical safety

☐ Store household cleaning products and other chemicals in a locked cabinet.

☐ Keep all vitamins and medications in a locked cabinet.

☐ Clearly label all chemicals and medications.

☐ Keep alcohol in a locked cabinet. Monitor and discourage alcohol use, because alcohol can increase confusion.

☐ Keep poison control phone numbers in a convenient location. Information for the national poison control center is provided in the Resources section at the end of this book.

## Checklist: Gun safety

☐ Remove firearms from the home; if this is not an option, lock the unloaded firearms in a gun safe to which your loved one does not have the key or combination.

☐ Lock bullets in a separate location from firearms. Bullets may present a choking hazard for individuals with Alzheimer's disease.

☐ Keep firearms unloaded when not in use.

## Medication Safety

Older adults, including individuals with Alzheimer's disease, often take a variety of medications for chronic diseases or conditions. Because of their deteriorating memory, individuals with Alzheimer's disease may forget to take their medication or may take the wrong dose. As a caregiver, one of your responsibilities will be to make sure your loved one takes the appropriate medications at the right doses on the schedule prescribed by the physician. Safety precautions related to medications are listed below.

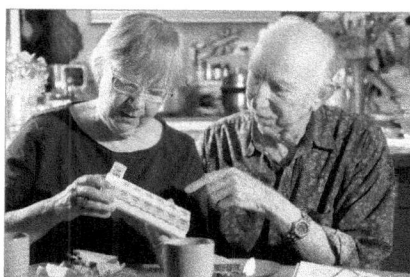

### *Checklist: Medication safety*

☐ Keep a complete and detailed list of your loved one's prescription medications, over-the-counter medications, vitamins, and herbal supplements with you at all times, including name, purpose, dose, and schedule.

☐ Discuss potential side effects and drug interactions with each of your loved one's healthcare providers.

☐ Keep a list of your loved one's drug allergies with you to discuss when receiving new medications.

☐ Supervise your loved one when taking medications to ensure the correct drug is taken at the correct time; this will help prevent overdosing or underdosing.

☐ If your loved one has a complex medication schedule, consider hiring a home health aide for one hour per day to make sure the medicine is taken properly.

☐ If your loved one has difficulty swallowing, ask the physician if there are other formulations of the medication your loved one can take, such as a liquid form. If you need to crush a pill, speak with the physician or pharmacist first, because some medications may become harmful or ineffective when crushed.

☐ If a physician has stated that medications can be mixed with food, mix those medications with soft foods such as applesauce or ice cream.

☐ Use a pill box organizer to plan your loved one's medication schedule.

☐ Develop a routine for giving medication to your loved one.

☐ Always provide clear, simple, step-by-step instructions to your loved one when taking medications.

☐ If your loved one won't take a medication, don't force them. Try again later.

## Wandering and Safety

Another important safety concern for individuals with Alzheimer's disease is wandering. Sixty percent of people with dementia will wander away from home at any time of the day or night or wander away from their loved ones when they are in public. Older adults with dementia who wander away from home often suffer serious injury or death if they are not found within the first 24 hours.

For caregivers, being able to recognize signs of wandering is an important first step for preventing wandering behavior. Wandering may be triggered by restlessness, anxiety, memory loss, disorientation, or physical needs such as hunger, thirst, or the urge to use the bathroom. Some warning signs are listed in the checklist below.

### *Checklist: Warning signs for wandering*

☐ Coming back from a drive or walk later than usual.

☐ Not being able to use keys or understand their purpose.

☐ Wanting to go home, even when they are at home.

☐ Having a hard time remembering their name or address.

☐ Getting off at the wrong stop when taking public transportation.

☐ Trying to go to work even though they are no longer working.

☐ Talking about going to a favorite location from the past that is not near their home.

☐ Asking where current or past family and friends are.

- [ ] Searching for a person or item that was lost at one time in the past.

- [ ] Restlessness and excessive pacing.

- [ ] Acting nervous in public or crowded areas.

- [ ] Appearing lost in a new or changed environment.

- [ ] Appearing more confused in the early evenings (known as "sundowning").

- [ ] Becoming lost or disoriented easily, even in familiar surroundings.

- [ ] Appearing to be participating in a productive activity without actually getting anything done.

- [ ] Trying to escape from a perceived threat, such as a strange visitor. Note that in the later stages of disease, even people your loved one has known for many years may seem like strangers. In extreme cases, your loved one may even react violently to a perceived "intruder."

The likelihood of your loved one having at least one wandering episode is very high, even if you take every precaution to prevent wandering. Before this occurs, you should take several steps to be prepared for a wandering episode.

## Checklist: Wandering preparations

- [ ] Enroll your loved one in an emergency response program such as MedicAlert® + Safe Return® and ensure that your loved one wears the alert bracelet at all times.

- [ ] Consider investing in a GPS tracking system for your loved one.

- [ ] Place an identification card and explanation of your loved one's condition in a purse or wallet that they are likely to take with them when they wander.

- [ ] If your loved one frequently takes public transportation, provide them with a map that shows their common stops, including their home stop. Even if your loved one won't use the map, others who stop to help them will find it useful.

- [ ] Place ID labels in your loved one's clothing.

- [ ] Have several recent photos and a description of your loved one available.

☐ Keep a piece of your loved one's worn, unwashed clothing in a plastic bag to aid in canine searches. Replace the clothing item every month to keep the scent strong, and wear gloves when handling the clothing to prevent contaminating the item with your scent.

☐ Notify the police and other emergency personnel in your area that your loved one has Alzheimer's disease and may wander. Provide them with a description of your loved one and other important information, such as name, address, your contact information, medication details, health conditions, and allergies.

☐ Notify neighbors of your loved one's condition and ask them to contact you if they ever see your loved one wandering alone.

☐ Make a list of people that you can call for help.

☐ Obtain the contact information for your state's Silver Alert program. A website that lists the state Silver Alert programs is included in the Resources section.

My father wandered. Sometimes he would end up at a neighbor's house, peeking in their windows and scaring them. Other times, he ended up at local businesses. One owner of a Subway sandwich shop was kind enough to recognize Dad, drive him home, and call me. Other wandering cases do not turn out so well. Alzheimer's patients can wander and get hurt by cars or end up in the cold, freezing. Once your loved one starts wandering, you must have a plan in place for 24-hour care. Any 24-hour solution to wandering will be expensive, but you likely will not have a choice.

Preventing episodes of wandering should begin long before your loved one starts wandering. Keep in mind that your loved one may not only wander from home. They may also wander away from you in public places. Preventing wandering episodes is especially important in extreme weather, such as extreme cold in winter, extreme heat in summer, or during storms. In addition to the preparedness steps above, practical steps to prevent wandering episodes are included in the checklist below.

## Checklist: Wandering prevention tips

☐ Don't leave your loved one unsupervised in an unfamiliar place or alone at home.

☐ Make sure your loved one gets enough exercise; physical activity is as important for individuals with Alzheimer's disease as it is for any other older adult.

☐ Keep a regular schedule of supervised daily activities such as folding laundry, sweeping, and preparing dinner.

☐ Provide special, meaningful activities for your loved one to participate in during the day, such as visiting with friends or going for a walk.

☐ Provide a room free of clutter in which your loved one can safely pace.

☐ If your loved one appears restless, make sure all their basic needs are met, especially eating, drinking, and toileting. If their basic needs are met, engage them in physical activity such as going for a walk together or engage them in a favorite TV program or other activity. Reassure them and make them feel loved and appreciated.

☐ Monitor your loved one's wandering patterns, especially any behaviors or events that may indicate that wandering is likely to happen soon. When you identify these behaviors, distract your loved one with an activity or take care of any needs that may be prompting wandering behaviors.

☐ Reassure your loved one if they feel lost, disoriented, or abandoned. Use simple phrases to encourage them to stay home, such as "you don't need to go in to work today" or "we decided to stay here tonight." Do not try to convince them that their reality is incorrect, because this will enhance their agitation.

☐ Identify bathrooms and other common rooms with large signs to help your disoriented loved one find their way.

☐ Place locks high and low on the door, and install locks with different opening mechanisms. This keeps the locks out of your loved one's direct line of sight and increases the difficulty of opening the door.

☐ Camouflage doors by painting them the same color as the wall or covering them with a window hanging or cloth.

☐ Cover door knobs with a cloth the same color as the door or install child safety knob covers.

☐ Place "STOP," "CLOSED," or "DO NOT ENTER" signs on external doors.

☐ Install buzzers or alarms that sound when an outside door is opened. Make sure these are loud enough for you to hear when you are sleeping.

- ☐ Install safety locks on windows.

- ☐ Install motion detectors that will alert you when your loved one is moving around, especially at night.

- ☐ If your loved one tends to wander at night, make sure that important items such as a glass of water, eyeglasses, clock, source of light, tissues, and telephone are next to them by the bed.

- ☐ Keep coats, shoes, keys, hats, purses, and wallets out of sight, because many older individuals will not leave home without these items.

- ☐ Fence in the yard with a high wooden fence that does not have footholds for climbing. Use locked gates to prevent easy access.

- ☐ Cover swimming pools and restrict access to them so your loved one does not become injured or drown.

- ☐ Control access to house keys, car keys, and cash to eliminate nonwalking methods of wandering (cars, buses, etc.).

- ☐ Avoid busy places that may cause confusion, such as shopping malls.

- ☐ Consult with a physician to determine if medication can help reduce wandering or if any of your loved one's medications may induce wandering.

Again, even if you have taken every precaution to prevent wandering, your loved one may still wander away from home. If this occurs, following the step-by-step instructions below can help you find your loved one as quickly as possible.

### Checklist: Steps for searching for your loved one

- ☐ Search the immediate area for no more than 15 minutes. Check nearby businesses or parks that your loved one may visit frequently.

- ☐ If a quick search does not locate your loved one, call 911 or your local equivalent immediately.

- ☐ Call your list of friends, family, and neighbors who have offered to help you search for your loved one.

- ☐ Distribute information to the search party, including a photo and current information such as clothing, height, and weight. If the police have search dogs, provide them with a piece of your loved one's scented clothing.

- ☐ Pinpoint areas of danger and search there first. These areas may include bodies of water, dense foliage, steep terrain, bus stops, busy highways, or tunnels.

- ☐ Search in the direction of your loved one's dominant hand (i.e., are they right-handed or left-handed?). People tend to turn first in that direction.

- ☐ Search areas that are familiar to your loved one, such as a park, old work location, former home, church, or favorite store.

- ☐ If a thorough search of the surrounding area does not find your loved one, call your state's Silver Alert program.

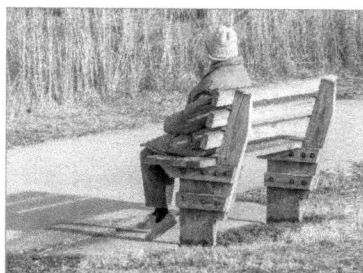

## Driving Safety

Impaired judgment, slowed reaction times, and impaired vision interpretation combine to make driving dangerous for individuals with Alzheimer's disease. However, a diagnosis of Alzheimer's disease does not automatically mean that your loved one can no longer drive safely. As a caregiver, you will need to observe your loved one's driving patterns to help discern when they need to give up driving, because all individuals with Alzheimer's disease will eventually reach a point when they no longer have the judgment and memory needed to drive safely.

Restricting or banning your loved one's driving privileges may result in tension and defiance, because they may interpret this action as taking away their independence. However, for the safety of your loved one and others on the road, you must stand firm when it is time to take the keys away. Taking my dad's keys away was one of the top-five worst days of my life. I hated doing something that was so hurtful to him and signified the end of his independence. Our relationship became so acrimonious as a result that I eventually told him I would give him his keys back if he passed the driving test at the Department of Motor Vehicles. I then printed off a practice written test and gave it to him. He never completed it, never gave it back to me, and we never spoke of his driving again.

The loss of driving abilities is inevitable for individuals with Alzheimer's disease. But how do you know that your loved one has gotten to the point of no longer being able to drive safely? The questions below can help you decide when it is appropriate to tell your loved one that they can no longer drive.

## Checklist: Is it safe for my loved one to be driving?

- ☐ Does your loved one understand the purpose of keys?

- ☐ Does your loved one know the difference between drive, reverse, and park?

- ☐ Can your loved one remember how to get to familiar places?

- ☐ Does your loved one forget where they are going during a trip?

- ☐ Can your loved one repeat their name, address, and phone number to a stranger when they are lost?

- ☐ Is your loved one slow to make decisions when driving?

- ☐ Is your loved one able to anticipate dangerous situations?

- ☐ Does your loved one have a shortened attention span?

- ☐ Is your loved one easily distracted while driving?

- ☐ Does your loved one become confused or angry while driving?

- ☐ Does your loved one become drowsy while driving?

- ☐ Does your loved one consistently obey traffic laws and signals?

- ☐ Has your loved one had a recent increase in accidents or traffic violations?

- ☐ Have you noticed any new dents or scratches on the car?

- ☐ Does your loved one drive at inappropriate speeds?

- ☐ Does your loved one appropriately use the gas and brake pedals?

- ☐ Does your loved one make spatial errors when driving, such as hitting the curb or wandering between lanes?

- ☐ Does your loved one have trouble negotiating turns, especially left-hand turns?

- ☐ Is your loved one able to park correctly?

- ☐ Do you feel safe riding in the car when your loved one is driving? Would you feel safe having your children ride with your loved one?

Once you have decided that you need to prevent your loved one from driving, how should you go about it? The discussion must be handled with care to avoid alienating or agitating your loved one. Consider some of the tips below when you are faced with this difficult discussion.

### Checklist: Tips for discussing driving limitations

- ☐ Have the discussion about driving long before your loved one is no longer able to drive to prepare them for this inevitable outcome. Involving your loved one in the decision process will help the transition go more smoothly.

- ☐ Recognize that you may need to have this discussion multiple times. For the person with Alzheimer's disease, it is better to have several short conversations than one long conversation.

- ☐ Discussions should be timed with other changes, such as changes in medication that may affect driving.

- ☐ Remember that a single instance of poor driving doesn't mean that your loved one should stop driving altogether. However, it does mean that your loved one should be monitored regularly for poor driving patterns.

- ☐ Document unsafe driving behaviors, and use them as evidence for why your loved one should no longer be driving.

- ☐ Avoid overreacting to driving incidents. Save the conversation about driving safety until after the immediate problem is resolved.

- ☐ Provide a simple explanation for why your loved one cannot drive. Focus on the disease rather than the individual as the reason to stop driving. Because thinking is slower for individuals with Alzheimer's disease, you may need to repeat the same simple sentence multiple times before they understand.

- ☐ Encourage your loved one to stop driving voluntarily. Appeal to your loved one's sense of responsibility to not endanger others on the road.

- [ ] Describe some advantages of no longer driving, such as saving money on gas, insurance, and car repairs.

- [ ] Acknowledge your loved one's feelings about losing the capability to drive, and confirm your unconditional love and support. Be patient but firm in your decision.

- [ ] Ask your loved one's physician to issue a "do not drive" prescription. Use the prescription to reinforce that they can no longer drive. Your loved one may take the news better coming from a doctor than from you or another friend or family member.

- [ ] Have your loved one take a driving test administered by the Department of Motor Vehicles. They should be tested at least annually until they are no longer able to drive.

If your loved one insists that they can still drive safely even though you and others have documented that they cannot, you may need to take drastic measures as a last resort to prevent your loved one from driving and endangering themselves and others. Some options for preventing your loved one from driving are included in the following checklist.

## Checklist: Driving prevention tips

- [ ] Control access to the car keys. If your loved one insists on carrying keys, provide them with old keys that do not work.

- [ ] Disable the car by removing the distributor cap or battery, or have a mechanic install a "kill switch" that must be flipped before the car will start.

- [ ] Keep the car out of sight or at a different location. This will help your loved one not think about driving as much.

- [ ] If you do not need the vehicle, consider selling your loved one's car and using the money to pay for other modes of transportation.

Although your loved one can no longer drive independently, they will still need to be transported to doctor's appointments, activities, and errands. Some solutions for making sure your loved one still has ready transportation are listed below.

## *Checklist: Alternative driving options*

- ☐ Slowly transition driving responsibilities to others. Alternative sources of transportation that are safe for your loved one can include family members or friends, a taxi service, or a special transportation service for older adults. Assisted living facilities also often provide group transportation services.

- ☐ Find ways to reduce your loved one's need to drive, such as having groceries and medications delivered.

- ☐ Tell your loved one that you are driving as a treat for them so they can sit back and enjoy the ride.

- ☐ When possible, walk with your loved one to your destination, and make it a special occasion

- ☐ Even if your loved one is no longer able to drive, they may be able to walk to neighboring businesses on their own to retain some independence. However, only allow them to walk in safe places that have sidewalks and slow traffic, and do not let them walk alone if they have a pattern of wandering or getting lost.

- ☐ When driving your loved one on errands, do not leave your loved one alone in a parked car.

## Disaster Safety

Disaster preparedness is one area of safety that is easy to overlook when caring for a loved one with Alzheimer's disease. However, if you live in an area that has frequent natural disasters, such as earthquakes, hurricanes, tornadoes, or forest fires, you need to have a plan in place to ensure your loved one's safety. Your loved one may not be able to recognize or respond to danger, may wander outside and get lost, or may not know how to get to a safe place before the disaster hits. Some ideas to help you and your loved one be prepared for a disaster are included in the checklist below.

## *Checklist: Disaster preparedness tips*

- ☐ Put together an emergency kit in a waterproof container and store it in a convenient location. The kit should include items such as copies of important documents and identification, extra medication and instructions, extra eyeglasses and hearing aid batteries, a recent picture of your loved one, basic first aid products, a flashlight with extra batteries, extra sets of clothing, incontinence products (if needed), bottled water, and favorite nonperishable food items. Different people have different needs, so consider your loved one's most basic needs and pack your emergency kit accordingly.

☐ Devise and practice an emergency exit plan. Make sure your emergency plan includes consideration of your loved one's specific needs, such as access to a walker or wheelchair. Update the plan frequently to reflect your loved one's changing capabilities.

☐ Assign one individual the responsibility of caring for your loved one during an emergency evacuation.

☐ When planning for a natural disaster or emergency, don't forget to include a plan for any pets your loved one has.

☐ Get to know your loved one's neighbors, and enlist them in helping you and your loved one during a natural disaster. Give neighbors important information such as contact information for caregivers, family members, and medical services. Teach them about your loved one's habits and struggles, and teach them how to provide simple instructions to your loved one.

☐ If your loved one lives in a long-term care facility, learn about the facility's emergency exit plan and find out who will be in charge of your loved one during the evacuation.

☐ Make sure your loved one always has an emergency alert bracelet on for identification.

☐ Write a plan for who will care for your loved one if something happens to you.

☐ Make an inventory of your loved one's possessions, and make sure they have adequate insurance coverage.

☐ Make your local law enforcement agency, fire department, emergency medical services, and hospitals aware of your loved one's condition. If an emergency occurs, they will know what to do if your loved one is confused.

☐ If you must go to a shelter or hotel for safety, make sure the staff knows about your loved one's condition.

☐ If you must evacuate to a hotel or shelter, use strategies to reduce your loved one's agitation such as taking a walk, talking calmly, or participating in an activity. Reassure your loved one that they are in the right place.

## Suicide Prevention

Even when every effort has been made to promote their independence and safety, some individuals with Alzheimer's disease contemplate or attempt suicide. These individuals fear losing the abilities to think, recognize their loved ones, and have meaningful interactions with the world around them. They also fear being a burden to their spouse, children, and friends based on their personal experiences with parents or others who had Alzheimer's disease. Suicide attempts often occur before the disease has progressed very far. In addition, there are many murder-suicide cases in which the healthy spouse kills their Alzheimer's-afflicted partner and then commits suicide. Some facts about suicide in patients with Alzheimer's disease and other forms of dementia are listed below.

### Checklist: Facts about Alzheimer's disease and suicide

☐ Individuals with a recent diagnosis of dementia are at higher risk for committing suicide, because they can still understand what the future may hold for them and their loved ones. The risk for suicide decreases as the disease progresses, because the individual loses the physical and mental capacity to commit suicide.

☐ Individuals with a history of depression and/or previous attempts to commit suicide are at higher risk of attempting suicide after a dementia diagnosis.

☐ Caucasians are more likely to commit suicide than other races, and men are more likely to commit suicide than women.

☐ A higher level of cognitive functioning is associated with an increased risk of suicide.

☐ The most common method of suicide is gunshot wound, which is why removing or locking guns is vitally important.

☐ If firearms are unavailable, individuals with dementia may overdose on drugs, hang themselves, or jump from a height to commit suicide.

☐ Individuals in full-time care facilities are less likely to commit suicide, probably because of the increased monitoring and more advanced disease stage.

As caregiver to a loved one with early stage Alzheimer's, how do you know if your loved one is contemplating suicide? Some warning signs are listed below.

### Checklist: Warning signs of suicide

☐ Your loved one exhibits the classic signs of depression, including withdrawal, apathy, fatigue, irritability, sleep problems, and feelings of helplessness or hopelessness.

☐ Your loved one becomes more socially isolated than they were before their Alzheimer's diagnosis.

☐ Your loved one states that they would rather leave their money behind for their loved ones than spend it on a full-time care facility.

☐ Your loved one states that they would prefer death to being unable to care for themselves and being unable to recognize their loved ones.

☐ Your loved one discusses feeling like a burden. Many individuals will state that they intend to commit suicide before they decline as much as a parent or other loved one who suffered from Alzheimer's disease.

☐ Your loved one begins to plan what will happen after their death; they plan their funeral and start to give away prized possessions.

☐ Your loved one mentions that they are planning to commit suicide before they reach the advanced stages of the disease.

☐ Your loved one admits to having a plan for how they will commit suicide.

☐ Your loved one wants to discuss the right time for them to take their own life. Most individuals plan to live as long as possible but commit suicide before the dementia becomes too severe.

If your loved one shows any of the above signs, what should you do? There are many potential options when caring for a loved one with Alzheimer's disease who is threatening to commit suicide. A few options are listed below.

*Checklist: Responding to a suicidal loved one*

☐ Assess your loved one's situation. Do they live alone? Do they have a history of suicide attempts?

☐ Evaluate your loved one's ability to carry out their plan for suicide. Do they have both the physical and mental capacity to kill themselves? Do they have access to drugs or a firearm?

☐ Consult with other family members about your loved one's condition and plan a strategy as a team.

☐ Talk to your loved one about their suicidal thoughts. Affirm your loved one's feelings without implying that you want them to commit suicide.

☐ Develop a safety plan with your loved one. This will encourage your loved one to call you or a trusted friend or family member before harming themselves.

☐ Talk to a physician about your loved one's suicidal ideations. The physician may be able to prescribe a medication or suggest a counselor for your loved one.

☐ Decrease your loved one's time alone. If your loved one lives alone at home, increase the number of times someone checks on them throughout the day. If your loved one lives in a full-time care facility, notify the staff and suggest frequent checks on your loved one.

## Utilizing Home Services

Even with appropriate independence and safety modifications in place, you may find it beneficial to look into home service options while your loved one is still living at home. During the early stages of the disease, your loved one will likely not need medical services or help with personal care unless there are other preexisting conditions, but they may benefit from companion services or homemaker services. Companion services can be arranged for once a week or multiple times a week, as needed. Homemaker services provide help with cooking, cleaning, laundry, food shopping, and other similar tasks. Even if your loved one is independent enough to live at home, both of these services can be helpful to decrease loneliness

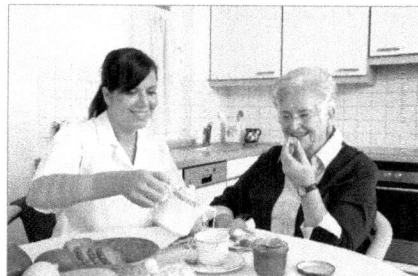

and frustration. To find local home service providers in your area, consult the Resources section at the end of the book. The checklist below discusses the duties performed by different home service providers.

## *Checklist: Types of duties performed by home services*

**Homemaker services:**

☐ Cooking

☐ Washing dishes

☐ Laundry

☐ Changing bed sheets

☐ Dusting

☐ Vacuuming

☐ Cleaning bathrooms

☐ Taking out trash

☐ Organization

☐ Medicine schedule reminders

☐ Pet care

☐ Houseplant care

☐ Errand assistance

☐ Grocery shopping

**Companion services:**

☐ Conversation

☐ Recreational activities (games, movies, walks, favorite hobbies, puzzles, etc.)

☐ Transportation to doctor's appointments or the grocery store

☐ Assistance in running errands

☐ Cognitive stimulation

- ☐ Help with phone calls

- ☐ Help with email or letter writing

- ☐ Light cleaning and cooking

**Personal care services:**

- ☐ Assistance with bathing

- ☐ Assistance with dressing

- ☐ Assistance with toileting

- ☐ Feeding assistance and monitoring

- ☐ Medicine reminders and monitoring

- ☐ Cooking

- ☐ Cleaning

- ☐ Laundry

- ☐ Changing bed sheets

- ☐ Shopping

- ☐ Providing transportation to appointments or the grocery store

Every Alzheimer's patient is unique in their needs and daily struggles. Therefore, there are no specific guidelines as to when your loved one will need different types of home services. The following checklist describes some indicators that your loved one may be in need of additional help around the house.

## Checklist: When should my loved one start receiving home services?

- ☐ Your loved one resists asking you for help with tasks around the house.

- ☐ The laundry is piling up without being washed.

- ☐ Your loved one wears clothes repeatedly without laundering them.

- ☐ Your loved one has not changed the bed sheets in weeks or has started sleeping on the couch because the bedding needs to be washed.

- ☐ The sink is always full of dirty dishes.

- ☐ You notice that many dishes are broken or misplaced.

- ☐ The refrigerator and cupboards have an abundance of expired and/or spoiled food.

- ☐ There is very little food in the house because your loved one has not gone grocery shopping.

- ☐ Your loved one is going without eating because they do not want to cook.

- ☐ Your loved one has a pet whose food dish is empty most times when you visit.

- ☐ Your loved one has difficulty bathing and/or dressing and is resistant to asking you or another family member for help.

- ☐ You notice that your loved one has bruises or injuries from falling when getting into or out of the shower or bathtub.

- ☐ Extra medication is present in your loved one's pill organizer because they have forgotten to take their pills multiple times.

- ☐ Unopened letters and correspondence pile up around the house.

- ☐ Your loved one's house has fallen well below the level of cleanliness your loved one maintained before becoming ill, and it is evident the home has not been vacuumed or dusted in weeks.

- ☐ Newspapers and other recyclables have started piling up.

- ☐ You realize that your loved one has very little social interaction and spends most days only watching television.

- ☐ The only person your loved one talks to most weeks is you.

- ☐ Your loved one frequently complains about feeling lonely.

- ☐ Your loved one is no longer able to drive but has various appointments during the day.

You do not need to arrange companion and homemaker services through an agency or outside source. A relative, family member, friend, or neighbor could stop by a few times a week to visit your loved one and help around the house. If you or your loved one has a large support network close by, such as friends, relatives, church companions, and/or community members, you can create a Caring Bridge website to set up a schedule of what everyone can do to help. (Please see the Resources section for more information.) This approach could ultimately relieve a lot of your stress. However, a large support group is not always available, so you also have the option to hire someone to perform these tasks. Both independent employees and caregiver service organizations are available; you can also sometimes find help through local churches, colleges with social work and nursing majors, senior centers, and community aid agencies. Before hiring someone for these positions, you should go through a thorough interview process. Consider the following checklist of questions when preparing for an interview.

### Checklist: Questions to ask when hiring companion and homemaker services

- ☐ What is the person's previous work experience?

- ☐ Have they worked with someone with Alzheimer's disease before?

- ☐ Will they submit to a background check?

- ☐ Do they have references?

- ☐ Have they ever been fired from a home service position before? If so, what was the reason for termination?

- ☐ In order to ensure they get along well with your loved one, are they willing to be hired on a trial basis first?

- ☐ Would your loved one prefer someone of the same gender to provide care, especially if they will be helping with bathing or dressing?

- ☐ Do they seem responsible? Have they answered all phone calls and/or emails in a timely manner? Did they show up to the interview on time?

- ☐ Do they have an agreeable personality/attitude?

- ☐ Do they appear to be patient?

- ☐ If they are interviewing to be a companion, what activities do they plan to do?

☐ Can they adjust their cooking style to meet the dietary needs of your loved one?

☐ Are they CPR and/or first aid certified?

☐ If they are applying to a position in which they will be driving your loved one, how is their driving record?

☐ Do they have a reliable form of transportation? Do they have car insurance?

☐ If they are applying for a position in which they will be expected to clean, are there any tasks they will not do? For example, are they opposed to cleaning toilets or washing dishes by hand?

## Utilizing Home Healthcare

Once your loved one progresses to the middle to late stages of Alzheimer's disease, they will likely need home healthcare services. Home healthcare could also be beneficial to your loved one in the earlier stages of the disease, especially if they have a preexisting condition or have difficulty taking medications properly. Home healthcare services are generally provided by a nurse or physician's assistant. This person can help with administering medications, bathing, eating, and sometimes even physical therapy. Home healthcare can be provided in your loved one's home as often as they need the services. The aide can visit weekly, daily, or even provide 24-hour-a-day care. If around-the-clock service is provided, this will generally allow your loved one to stay in their home longer, avoiding the need to move in with a caregiver.

### Checklist: When to hire home healthcare

☐ Your loved one needs help with medications.

☐ Your loved one needs wound care.

☐ Your loved one is experiencing medical problems beyond your care abilities, especially medical problems in addition to Alzheimer's disease (e.g., diabetes, heart disease, or blood clots).

☐ Your loved one needs daily or weekly injections.

☐ Your loved one gets infections easily.

☐ Your loved one requires specialized medical equipment.

☐ You are making frequent visits to the doctor for things that could be handled by a nurse at your loved one's home.

☐ Your loved one has particular diet and nutritional needs.

☐ Your loved one needs help bathing and dressing.

☐ Your loved one requires physical therapy.

Before hiring someone to work with your loved one, you should do some research into the company or service you are considering. Some resources to help with this research are included at the end of the book. The following checklist also discusses what to look for when hiring home healthcare.

*Checklist: What to look for when hiring home healthcare*

☐ Does the healthcare service run background checks on its employees?

☐ Are the employees trained to care for patients with Alzheimer's disease?

☐ What kind of training do the employees receive?

☐ What skill level are the employees? RNs? CNAs?

☐ How are the employees monitored to ensure a high quality of care?

☐ What policies are in place to handle problems if they arise?

☐ Will you be able to personally choose/interview the employees who will be working with your loved one?

☐ Will the service accept patients who are incontinent?

☐ Can the home healthcare worker take your loved one to the hospital if necessary, or will an ambulance need to be called?

☐ Will the worker wait with your loved one until you get to the hospital?

☐ Will you need to provide meals for the home healthcare worker, or will they bring their own?

☐ Is it possible to do a trial day/week to see how the employee and your loved one interact together?

☐ Will your loved one be assigned a regular healthcare worker, or will the person change each day/week?

☐ If a regular healthcare worker is not available to come due to illness or other factors, will a replacement be sent? If so, how will you be notified of the replacement?

☐ How long has the company been in business?

☐ What kind of reputation does the company have within the community?

☐ Is the service only available during the week, or do they have weekend care as well?

☐ Is the company an approved Medicare or Medicaid provider?

☐ Does the company honor the Patient's Bill of Rights (i.e., the patient's overall rights in terms of care, such as being treated with respect)?

☐ Will the company provide you with a sample plan of care for a client with Alzheimer's disease?

☐ What is the company's policy on patient confidentiality?

☐ Are fees fixed, or do they work on a sliding scale?

☐ Is financial assistance available when needed?

☐ Is the company licensed by the state?

☐ Do the company's representatives seem friendly and helpful?

☐ Does the company have relationships with dietitians, counselors, and/or other specialists? Can they provide referrals if/when they are needed?

☐ How quickly can services begin?

## Employing a Geriatric Care Manager

When you feel it is time to hire home services, consider finding a geriatric care manager who will oversee your loved one's home care. Geriatric care managers are generally social workers, counselors, nurses, or other professionals in the field of geriatrics (a branch of medicine specializing in the care of older adults). The role of a geriatric care managers to aid families and their loved ones with the many challenges associated with finding appropriate care. For your loved one with Alzheimer's disease, a care manager would get to know your loved one as well as the family, then work to suggest the best possible care in terms of insurance, resources, and the reputation of the facility, if applicable. These managers help to facilitate care, whether in the home or in a residential facility. If, as a caregiver, you are overwhelmed by determining the best living arrangements for your loved one, or you are unsure if your loved one's current living arrangements are in their best interest, then you may want to consider a geriatric care manager.

Geriatric care managers are rarely, if ever, covered by insurance companies or Medicare, and their fees may prohibit you from considering this option. However, a sliding scale fee can sometimes be arranged depending on the company or individual being hired. If you are interested in this type of service, conduct research to find an agency that provides the services you want at the best price. The checklists below discuss the services that most geriatric care managers offer, signs to help you determine which services might be useful, and what to look for in a care manager.

### Checklist: What services do geriatric care managers provide?

- ☐ Customize all services and suggestions specifically to your loved one's needs by performing in-depth interviews with caregivers, family, and your loved one.

- ☐ Recommend a care plan tailored to your loved one's needs.

- ☐ Set up and attend doctor's appointments with your loved one.

- ☐ Ensure communication between doctors and your loved one and family.

- ☐ Act as an advocate for you and your loved one in cases where there are disagreements with a living facility, hospital, or doctor.

- ☐ Manage your loved one's medication schedule.

- ☐ Help plan for your loved one's future needs based on the progression of their disease.

- ☐ Help avoid preventable or unnecessary hospitalization, incorrect placements, and/or duplicated services.

- ☐ Suggest the most appropriate forms of home care services needed.

- ☐ Suggest measures that can be taken to make your loved one's environment safer as their disease progresses.

- ☐ Recommend and facilitate social and recreational activities.

- ☐ Monitor your loved one's condition and suggest changes in housing arrangements and/or services when necessary.

- ☐ Help select living arrangements, organize all details to facilitate the move, and smooth the transition between living situations.

- ☐ Provide crisis intervention and counseling, as needed.

- ☐ Recommend legal assistance by working with elder care attorneys. (See *Advance Directives, Durable Power of Attorney, Wills, and Other Legal Considerations* for more information.)

- ☐ Facilitate management of finances by working closely with the individual to whom your loved one has given power of attorney.

- ☐ Monitor your loved one's well-being, watching for signs of emotional, physical, and/or financial abuse.

- ☐ Alert family and caregivers to any problems.

## Checklist: Signs you might need a geriatric care manager

- ☐ Your loved one has no family members nearby and you are trying to manage care from another state.

- ☐ You and/or your loved one are confused regarding housing arrangements as the disease progresses.

- ☐ The environment your loved one is currently living in is unsafe, but you do not know how to fix the situation.

- ☐ You and/or your family are burned out and unsure what care decisions would be best.

- ☐ You have been trying to research living arrangements, medical needs, and other care-related elements for Alzheimer's disease, but you are confused and frustrated.

- ☐ You are having difficulty communicating your loved one's needs to the facility where they are currently living.

- ☐ Your relationship with the facility where your loved one is currently living has become hostile and/or increasingly strained.

- ☐ Your family disagrees about the best course of action regarding care decisions and living arrangements.

- ☐ You and/or your loved one have many questions regarding financial and legal matters.

- ☐ Your loved one is in need of a strong care advocate.

- ☐ You and/or your family feel they would benefit from further education about changes that will need to be made as your loved one's disease progresses.

- ☐ Your loved one has become violent and/or withdrawn and depressed.

## *Checklist: What to look for when hiring a geriatric care manager*

### Geriatric care management company:

- ☐ How long has the company been providing this service?

- ☐ Are the care managers trained to work with individuals who have Alzheimer's disease?

- ☐ What kind of training do the care managers receive?

- ☐ Will the company provide references for care managers?

- ☐ Do all employees undergo a background check?

- ☐ What types of backgrounds do the company's geriatric care managers have (e.g. social work, nursing, or counseling)?

- ☐ How does the company supervise its care managers?

- ☐ How often will you be updated about your loved one's situation?

- ☐ How much does the company charge for a consultation?

- ☐ How much do they charge for services?

- ☐ Do they offer sliding scale fees?

- ☐ Do they offer the services you need most?

- ☐ Can the company show you an example of a care plan they have used for a client with Alzheimer's disease?

- ☐ Are care managers available on weekends and holidays?

**Independent geriatric care managers:**

- ☐ How long has the individual been offering geriatric care management services?

- ☐ How many clients has the individual worked with to date?

- ☐ Have any of these clients had Alzheimer's disease? If so, how many?

- ☐ Has the individual received training to work with individuals with Alzheimer's disease?

- ☐ Will the individual submit to a background check?

- ☐ Will the individual provide a list of references?

- ☐ What is the person's background (e.g., nursing, social work, or counseling)?

- ☐ Is the individual a certified geriatric care manager?

- ☐ Is the person familiar with the resources and overall area in which your loved one lives?

- ☐ How often will you be updated on your loved one's case?

- ☐ How much does the individual charge for services?

- ☐ How many other clients will the person have in addition to your loved one? Or will your loved one be the person's primary client?

- ☐ Is the individual friendly and approachable?

- ☐ Do you like the person? Do you think you could trust and work with this person over the long term?

- ☐ Does the individual seem responsible? Has the person answered your phone calls and/or emails in a timely manner?

- ☐ Can the individual provide examples of care plans that they have drawn up for other clients with Alzheimer's disease?

- ☐ Does the person offer the services you need most?

- ☐ Is the person in contact with an elder care attorney? Or does the person have a strong knowledge of elder care laws?

- ☐ Is the individual available for emergencies?

- ☐ Does the person provide consultation on weekends and holidays, if necessary?

- ☐ Does the person belong to any professional organizations in their field?

# Leaving Home

Many individuals with Alzheimer's disease should not be left at home alone, especially in the advanced stages of the disease. Even if your loved one has been able to remain at home thanks to the help of visiting service providers, a time will come when you notice their condition is worsening. You will become aware of greater difficulties and dangerous situations your loved one is experiencing. You may even find it almost impossible to relax or sleep through the night because you are constantly worried about your loved one's safety. These are all signs that you should reassess your loved one's living situation. The following checklist highlights some signs that, either individually or in combination, could indicate it is no longer safe for your loved one to live alone.

### Checklist: Signs it is no longer safe for your loved one to live alone

- ☐ Your loved one has difficulty walking independently.

- ☐ Your loved one has experienced a few instances of wandering.

- ☐ Your loved one has difficulty repeating their phone number and address.

- ☐ Your loved one has demonstrated warning signs for suicide.

- ☐ Your loved one has presented fire safety concerns, such as trying to cook but leaving the stove on or ignoring the smoke detectors.

- ☐ Your loved one gets confused or scared easily in their own house.

- [ ] Your loved one becomes easily confused when under stress.

- [ ] Your loved one needs someone around 24 hours a day.

- [ ] Your loved one is scared to be alone.

- [ ] Your loved one is having difficulty successfully bathing or dressing.

- [ ] Your loved one has had a few minor falls and/or a more severe fall that caused injuries.

- [ ] Your loved one is becoming increasingly withdrawn and/or depressed.

- [ ] Your loved one has difficulty eating or swallowing.

- [ ] Weight loss has become apparent because your loved one has stopped eating.

- [ ] Your loved one frequently appears restless.

- [ ] Your loved one has difficulty using the phone.

- [ ] Your loved one's ability to communicate has begun declining rapidly.

- [ ] Your loved one's hygiene difficulties have become apparent, such as not bathing, forgetting to brush their teeth or hair, and wearing the same clothes each day.

- [ ] Your loved one has stopped taking medication properly.

- [ ] You feel that your loved one would not know what to do in case of an emergency, such as a fire, power outage, injury, or illness.

## Managing the Moving Process

When the time comes for your loved one to leave home, the change in surroundings will likely cause them a great deal of stress. No matter what stage of Alzheimer's disease your loved one is in, moving can be especially hard. However, this is particularly true for individuals in the later stage of Alzheimer's disease.

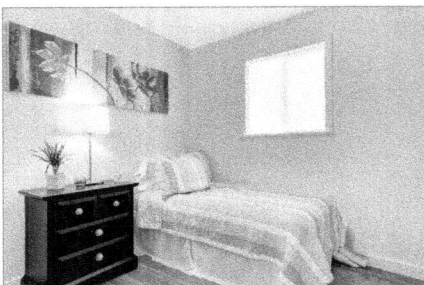

Major moves should be planned well in advance, if possible, in order to ensure the best acclimation to the new environment. If your loved one becomes stressed as a result of moving, their behaviors may become more difficult to manage; alternatively, your loved one could become more withdrawn. Both reactions are entirely normal, as long as they begin to subside in a reasonable amount of time. Keep in mind that acclimating to a new environment does not occur overnight for an individual with Alzheimer's disease. Sometimes it could take your loved one two to three weeks to become comfortable with their new living environment. Depending on how severe your loved one's reaction to the move is, you and other family members may have to avoid visiting for a time to allow your loved one to get used to the new surroundings. This can be difficult for you, and most facilities will allow you to look in on your loved one so that you know they are safe and well, but without your loved one being able to actually see you. In addition, a number of steps can be taken to ensure that the move and subsequent transition are as smooth as possible.

## *Checklist: Easing the transition*

- ☐ Bring your loved one to the new residence a few times before they move in.

- ☐ Talk to the caregivers or staff about your loved one's habits, favorite foods, preferred activities, etc.

- ☐ Inform the caregivers or staff about any daily rituals or schedules your loved one generally follows.

- ☐ Decorate your loved one's room before the move-in day.

- ☐ Bring familiar pictures, blankets, quilts, and decorations for your loved one's new room.

- ☐ If your loved one has a favorite chair or piece of furniture, consider bringing it for their room.

- ☐ Put together scrapbooks or photo albums with pictures of loved ones, and make sure to label the pictures with names.

- ☐ Decorate the walls with family photos.

- ☐ Move items from your loved one's old home to the new residence when your loved one is not around

☐ Be positive during the move and when talking to your loved one about the new place.

☐ If moving to a care facility, have at least two people accompany your loved one on move-in day; this way, one person can fill out any paperwork and talk to the staff while the other person stays with your loved one.

☐ When you leave, try not to make a big production; instead, slip away quietly.

☐ Recognize that it will take a few weeks for your loved one to become acclimated to the new surroundings.

☐ If your loved one becomes agitated or stressed when you visit in the first few weeks, consider limiting your visits in order to ease their transition.

# Moving in with a Caregiver

When your loved one can no longer remain home alone, there are several types of living arrangements to consider. One option is for your loved one to move in with a caregiver, while another is for a caregiver to move into your loved one's home. With both of these options, caregivers are usually children or close relatives of individuals with Alzheimer's disease.

Choosing to share a home with their loved one is the first alternative many people consider, but it is not the correct choice for everyone. Before making a decision, you need to find the option that works best for you and your family. Consider the checklists below to determine whether having your loved one move in with you is a good option.

### Checklist: Should my loved one move in with me?

☐ Can my loved one safely live alone?

☐ Do I have extra room in my house for my loved one?

☐ Do I have the monetary resources to hire someone to be with my loved one during the day, or can I be home during the day with my loved one?

☐ Is this option more affordable than a live-in facility?

☐ Can I handle the emotional stress?

- ☐ Can my children/spouse handle the emotional stress?

- ☐ Will my job situation allow for me to leave at a moment's notice to take care of emergencies that will inevitably occur while my loved one lives at home?

- ☐ Have my loved one and I decided this should be the next step before considering an independent or full-time living facility?

- ☐ Do I have relief care options in place to avoid becoming burned out?

- ☐ Do I want full control over the care my loved one receives?

- ☐ Would I feel safer if my loved one was not living at home alone?

- ☐ Do my loved one and I one get along well with each other? If you and your loved one do not communicate well in low-stress situations, then it is likely that moving them into your home will create unnecessary stress for both of you.

- ☐ Can I be patient with my loved one when they get frustrated or have a bad day?

- ☐ Is my loved one violent?

- ☐ Can my home be easily (and affordably) converted to meet the progressive needs of my loved one?

- ☐ Does my loved one need around-the-clock, skilled medical attention?

- ☐ Can my loved one eat on their own?

### Checklist: Pros and cons of moving in with a caregiver

**Pros:**

- ☐ It is less expensive than a residential facility.

- ☐ Your loved one is close by.

- ☐ Your loved one will be in a familiar environment.

- ☐ You will be able to easily spend more time with your loved one.

- ☐ You will have more control over the type of care being received.

- ☐ You will be more involved with your loved one's medical care.

- ☐ You can ensure your loved one gets daily exercise and cognitive stimulation.

☐ You will have more control over the visitors your loved one receives.

☐ You will be able to monitor for fraud and scams more easily.

**Cons:**

☐ Caregivers have a high chance of burnout.

☐ Caring for an individual who is losing their memory can be extremely stressful.

☐ Being a primary caregiver is time consuming.

☐ Your sleeping, eating, and daily habits will have to change to accommodate your loved one's habits.

☐ Your daily routines could be disrupted, particularly if you have young children.

☐ You will be responsible for your loved one's safety and well-being.

☐ As the disease progresses, it may become harder to be the primary caregiver.

☐ Your loved one may eventually have to be moved to a residential facility.

☐ You will need to hire home healthcare services.

Before deciding to have your loved one move in with you and your family, you should know the duties and responsibilities you will have. Live-in caregivers to individuals with Alzheimer's disease often become burned out because they do not understand the amount of work, and sometimes stress, that comes with this role. For example, in the United States in 2014 alone, more than 15 million caregivers provided roughly 17.9 billion hours of care to individuals with Alzheimer's disease. Collectively, this care was valued at approximately $217.7 billion. Therefore, taking on the role of live-in caregiver is a momentous decision. The following checklist discusses some of the responsibilities you will have if your loved one moves into your home.

## Checklist: What are the roles of a live-in caregiver?

☐ Implement a daily routine.

☐ Plan nutritious, healthy meals.

☐ Prepare medications, monitor whether they are taken correctly, and watch for signs of adverse medication reactions.

☐ Organize daily physical activities and exercise, as well as daily activities to engage the mind.

☐ Ensure your loved one has opportunities for socializing and plan visits with friends and family.

☐ Plan activities to keep your loved one from sitting around most of the day.

☐ Organize your loved one's participation in spiritual activities, if this is something they have always done or they want to do.

☐ Monitor holiday celebrations, and your loved one's reaction to these events, to prevent anxiety and stress.

☐ Support your loved one when they become discouraged, frustrated, or anxious.

☐ Prevent your loved one from experiencing too much stress. (High stress will speed progression of the disease and cause unnecessary anxiety.)

☐ Assist your loved one with bathing, dressing, and toileting when needed.

☐ Help your loved one with daily grooming, such as brushing their teeth, cleaning their dentures, shaving, cleaning their fingernails, etc.

☐ Stay patient and calm when helping your loved one.

☐ Work to ensure your loved one's safety in the home, as well as out in public.

☐ Assess and modify the house for safety as your loved one's illness progresses.

☐ Watch for signs of wandering and sundowning.

☐ Prevent your loved one from wandering, especially at night when you could be sleeping.

☐ Ensure that your loved one is getting enough sleep.

☐ Arrange doctor and specialist appointments, as well as transportation to those appointments.

☐ Act as an advocate for your loved one with doctors, and potentially even other family members. (This is primarily the responsibility of a healthcare agent.)

☐ Monitor your loved one for signs of advancing cognitive deterioration.

☐ Watch for significant changes in your loved one's personality and/or communication skills.

☐ Manage, or help manage, your loved one's finances. (This is primarily the responsibility of a durable power of attorney for finances.)

☐ Hire home services (home healthcare, homemaker, and/or companion services) when they are needed.

Helping your loved one maintain independence is important when they move in with you, because increased independence can be beneficial to their overall well-being. The checklist below discusses some tips for helping your loved one maintain their independence after the move.

### Checklist: Tips for maintaining independence when living with a caregiver

☐ Try not to be overprotective and do everything for your loved one. They can likely still help in many ways.

☐ Encourage your loved one to participate in decisions about their health, activities, and options whenever possible.

☐ Give your loved one as much freedom in the house as possible.

☐ If your loved one is having difficulty performing a particular task, offer to help but do not take over or do the task for them.

☐ Encourage your loved one to help around the house with small tasks such as setting the table, washing dishes, folding laundry, etc.

☐ Have your loved one help you prepare a meal they used to cook regularly.

☐ Ask your loved one to help with baking, if that is something they once enjoyed.

☐ Ask for your loved one's opinion on cooking; maybe have them taste the food and offer suggestions. (Note: As the disease progresses, your loved one may begin to lose their sense of smell and taste.)

☐ Make sure to give your loved one choices. If they become anxious due to having too many options, limit choices to two things. For example, ask your loved one if they would like meatloaf or soup for dinner.

☐ If you have children, encourage your loved one to help with them. Being around children can be a low-stress situation for individuals with Alzheimer's disease, because they are less likely to feel as though they are being judged. It could also help bring back good memories of your loved one's childhood.

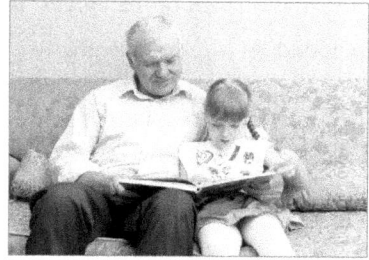

☐ Ask your loved one to help care for your pet (if you have one). Your loved one could help take the pet for walks (with someone's company if they are prone to wandering) or help feed the animal. Pets can be very therapeutic.

☐ Encourage your loved one to help you with gardening or taking care of indoor plants, if that was something they once enjoyed. Ensure that none of the plants are poisonous if ingested, and always stay with your loved when using tools in the garden that could lead to injury.

☐ Plan outings once a week if your loved one is able, and give them a choice of the location.

☐ If your loved one has stopped participating in hobbies or activities because the illness has made it difficult, offer to participate in those activities together. For example, you could go for walks together at night or work on a craft your loved one enjoys.

☐ If your loved one has started to have incontinence problems, do not make a big deal out of it. Buy disposable underwear and leave them in the bathroom your loved one uses; tell your loved one where you placed the underwear, but do not mention it again unless necessary.

## Caregiver Agreements

When your loved one is unable to provide their own care, a family member often steps in to become caregiver. Sometimes, the caregiver goes to your loved one's home for several hours each day to provide care. In other situations, the caregiver may move in with your loved one or your loved one may move in with the caregiver, as discussed above. This can create both financial and emotional hardship for the caregiver, especially if the caregiver is required to give up a steady job with benefits to provide care. If one individual is providing the majority of care for your loved one, your family may want to create a caregiver agreement that allows your loved one to pay the caregiver for the care they provide. The following checklists provide basic information about caregiver agreements as well as information that should be included in these agreements. For sample care agreements, see the links in the Resources section.

## Checklist: Basics about a caregiver agreement

☐ A caregiver agreement is a contract between an ill individual and a caregiver that lists caregiving responsibilities and compensation for care provided. It may also be called a personal care agreement, long-term care personal support services agreement, elder care contract, family care contract, or caregiver contract.

☐ A caregiver agreement can be used to compensate a family member who has made a great personal sacrifice in order to provide care for a loved one. This prevents the caregiver from experiencing undue financial hardship due to their caregiving responsibilities.

☐ A caregiver agreement is used to stipulate payment for future caregiving services. It should not provide compensation for past caregiving services.

☐ A caregiving agreement can help prevent family conflicts over who should provide care and what type of care they should provide.

☐ The caregiver agreement should be put in writing. This allows the caregiver and family members to have a record of the caregiver's responsibilities and compensation, as well as to provide proof to Medicaid and other government assistance programs that the transfer of money between your loved one and the caregiver was for caregiving services and not a gift. (See *Long-Term Care Insurance, Power of Attorney, Wealth Management, and Other First Steps* for more information about Medicare eligibility and gifts.) Because a caregiving agreement may affect the inheritance, all family members should help construct the agreement, especially the amount the caregiver will be compensated.

☐ A caregiver agreement provides your loved one with peace of mind that they will be cared for when they are no longer able to provide their own care.

☐ A lawyer is not needed to complete a caregiver agreement, but it may be beneficial to consult a lawyer for complicated agreements.

## *Checklist: Characteristics of a caregiver*

☐ Often an adult child of the individual with Alzheimer's disease, although adult grandchildren, other relatives, or friends may also provide care.

☐ Should live close to your loved one with Alzheimer's disease.

☐ Should be someone your loved one knows, not a stranger.

☐ Often has few personal responsibilities, such as no minor children living at home.

☐ Should be willing to give up a paying job if necessary to care for your loved one, provided they will be paid for providing care to your loved one.

☐ Willing to take on the enormous time commitment and responsibility associated with caring for a loved one with Alzheimer's disease.

☐ Responsible and even-tempered.

☐ Understands the list of responsibilities and how to perform the needed tasks.

## *Checklist: Information to include in a caregiver agreement*

☐ The date care should begin. For individuals with Alzheimer's disease, this may be a vague date in the future based on the progression of the disease.

☐ How long the agreement is in effect (e.g., one year, five years, or for the lifetime of the ill individual).

☐ A detailed description of care to be provided. You may want to have a care assessment conducted in the home or consult your loved one's medical records to help determine the care needed. Specifically defining the care tasks to be completed and the time they will take will help compensation and time expectations be more reasonable.

☐ Provisions for expanded responsibilities as your loved one's disease progresses.

☐ A description of where the care will take place (e.g., at your loved one's home or in the caregiver's home). Allow for a change of location as needed based on your loved one's stage of disease.

☐ How many hours of caregiving will be provided each week. For individuals with Alzheimer's disease, the number of caregiving hours may need to be given on a sliding scale based on the progression of the disease. Language should allow for flexibility, such as "up to 20 hours per week" or "no less than 160 hours per month."

☐ The amount of compensation for the caregiver. Compensation for care should be similar to what the family would pay a third party to provide care. The family may need to do some research into the amount they would pay a caregiving service for a similar level of care. The amount of compensation should reflect the complexity of caregiving duties and the time spent on caregiving duties.

☐ When the caregiver will be compensated (e.g., weekly, biweekly, monthly).

☐ Provisions for raises in the future to compensate for a job well done.

☐ Provisions for living expense compensation (e.g., room and board, utilities) if your loved one lives with the caregiver; also make sure that homeowners insurance covers liabilities such as work injuries.

☐ Provisions for health insurance and other benefits for the caregiver, especially if they resigned from a job with benefits to provide care for your loved one.

☐ Your loved one's responsibility versus the caregiver's responsibility for paying withholding taxes and Social Security.

☐ Provisions for incidental out-of-pocket expenses, including but not limited to home modifications for safety.

☐ A statement of who will write the caregiver's paychecks. This should be your loved one's power of attorney for finances; if the caregiver is also the power of attorney, consult a trustee or other legal representative.

☐ If the caregiver will be responsible for transportation, stipulations regarding the level of car insurance that is needed.

☐ Provisions for respite time or vacation time for the caregiver.

- ☐ Provisions for caregiving backup if the caregiver goes on vacation, gets sick, or needs respite time.

- ☐ A statement that the agreement can be modified only by mutual agreement of both parties. Any modifications should be put in writing and signed and dated by both parties.

- ☐ A statement that the caregiver can void the contract if the caregiving duties exceed their abilities. For example, a caregiver may feel unqualified to care for your loved one in the final stages of Alzheimer's disease.

- ☐ Signatures of both parties and the date. If your loved one is not legally competent to sign the document, their durable power of attorney for finances or conservator can sign for them. If the caregiver and your loved one's legal financial representative are the same person, consider consulting an attorney.

### Checklist: Types of caregiver duties listed in a caregiver agreement

- ☐ Hygiene care (e.g., bathing, dressing, grooming)

- ☐ Nutrition (e.g., cooking, special diet considerations, feeding, grocery shopping)

- ☐ Mobility (e.g., assisting with transfers from the bed to a chair)

- ☐ Monitoring medications

- ☐ Tracking changes in health

- ☐ Companionship

- ☐ Monitoring for safety (e.g., wandering, driving, home safety, medication safety)

- ☐ Housekeeping (e.g., cleaning, laundry, dishes, errands); may list individual tasks if needed

- ☐ Outdoor maintenance (e.g., mowing lawn, trimming bushes, raking leaves, snow removal)

- ☐ Financial tasks (e.g., paying bills and balancing the checkbook); note that this may be the duty of a power of attorney rather than the caregiver

- ☐ Car maintenance (e.g., taking your loved one's car to the shop for oil changes)

- [ ] Transportation to appointments and events; consider mileage when establishing compensation

- [ ] Consulting with physicians and other medical personnel; note that this may be the duty of a healthcare agent rather than the caregiver

- [ ] Creating a daily log of activities; this will help with Medicare or other documentation as well as provide evidence of services provided

- [ ] Recording payment of expenses for government assistance documentation

## Caregiver Burnout

If you are your loved one's primary caregiver, you may suffer the effects of caregiver burnout over time. Caregiver burnout occurs due to the accumulation of stress and responsibility that the caregiver experiences. If your loved one moves in with you, a routine will likely develop. However, as the disease progresses into the middle and later stages, this routine will probably become more and more complicated, which will ultimately leave you with more responsibility and less time for yourself. The signs of caregiver burnout are gradual, but you need to watch for them in order to avoid later complications. Being aware of the signs will also enable you to work toward reversing the effects. The following checklist discusses the signs of caregiver burnout.

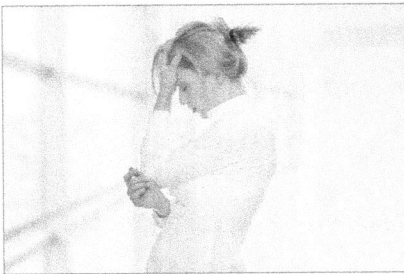

### Checklist: Signs of caregiver burnout

- [ ] You feel more overwhelmed than usual.

- [ ] You do not exercise or relax because you feel that there is no time.

- [ ] Your anxiety levels have started increasing.

- [ ] You have lost your temper with a loved one because they are not responding the way you want or expect.

- [ ] You are yelling at and/or becoming angry with coworkers, loved ones, and friends for no reason.

- ☐ Your emotions change quickly and drastically (e.g., you are angry one minute and extremely sad the next).

- ☐ You are not sleeping well due to stress or anxiety.

- ☐ You find that you are exhausted all the time.

- ☐ You are frequently giving up social and family events.

- ☐ You haven't spent time with friends or engaged in leisure activities in months.

- ☐ You no longer enjoy activities you once favored.

- ☐ You feel that you are unable to give your loved one the help they need.

- ☐ Your weight or appetite has changed.

- ☐ You have been ill more often than usual.

- ☐ You are having trouble concentrating on tasks.

- ☐ You are having difficulty remembering appointments or events.

- ☐ You have had thoughts of suicide.

- ☐ You have had thoughts about hurting your loved one.

- ☐ You find yourself wishing it would all be over so that your stress could end.

If you think you might be suffering from caregiver burnout, seek help for yourself and assistance with your caregiving responsibilities. Numerous support groups exist where you can meet with other people in your area who are experiencing similar difficulties. (Please see the Resources section for help finding support groups near you.) If you need a break from caregiver duties, consider taking a short vacation or having family members or a service come in one or two afternoons a week to give you time for yourself. The checklist below discusses some options for services that could help give you a break from your caregiver duties.

### Checklist: Respite care and adult day care

**Respite care:**

- ☐ Respite care provides you with a few hours to get out of the house and have some time to yourself.

- ☐ It occurs in your home, so your loved one would not have to leave.

- ☐ It gives your loved one a chance to interact with another person.

- ☐ It can offer you extra time to do errands.

- ☐ It helps prevent caregiver burnout.

- ☐ Friends, family, or neighbors can provide respite care.

- ☐ Community organizations offer respite care services.

- ☐ You can hire services such as homemaker and companion services to provide respite care.

- ☐ Some residential facilities offer short-term stays for respite care (one night to a few weeks).

**Adult day care:**

- ☐ Adult day care is a place where your loved one is cared for by trained staff while you are at work, running errands, or taking a needed break.

- ☐ You will be able to relax knowing that your loved one is safe and cared for.

- ☐ Transportation is sometimes provided to and from the day care facility.

- ☐ Adult day care is offered in a location outside of your home.

- ☐ Most centers are open between seven and ten hours a day.

- ☐ Some facilities are open over the weekend and have evening hours.

- ☐ Most centers have social workers and nurses on staff.

- ☐ The staff is often trained to work with individuals who have dementia. Some adult day centers specialize in caring for individuals with Alzheimer's disease.

- ☐ These facilities supply nutritious meals and snacks throughout the day.

- ☐ You loved one can receive assistance with eating, when necessary.

- ☐ You loved one is provided with assistance taking medications during the day.

- ☐ Your loved one will engage in light physical exercise.

☐ Physical, occupational, and speech therapy may be offered at these facilities.

☐ These facilities often teach relaxation techniques.

☐ Many facilities offer pet therapy and music therapy, which can be beneficial.

☐ Your loved one is provided with activities to stimulate their mind.

☐ Your loved one will be able to interact with others and participate in social activities.

☐ Activities such as games, gardening, field trips, and crafts are planned throughout the day to keep your loved one entertained and active.

☐ Some facilities offer counseling for both your loved one and your family, if needed.

☐ Medicaid generally covers most, if not all, adult day care costs.

☐ Private insurance and long-term care insurance will sometimes cover the cost of adult day care.

## Moving to Assisted Living

Because of the immeasurable stress placed on the caregiver and the potential for caregiver burnout, having your loved one live at home alone or with a caregiver may not be a viable option in the later stages of the disease. If you decide that having your loved one move in with you is not a good choice for you and your family, consider an independent facility. Independent facilities are also referred to as assisted living facilities, adult living centers, and supported care facilities. These residences allow the individuals living there to have a greater sense of independence than they would experience in a hospital or nursing home, but the facility also provides assistance with day-to-day activities. Independent facilities do not offer around-the-clock skilled medical care. If this is needed, then you should consider a nursing home or other full-time care facility.

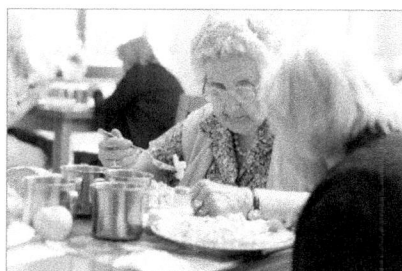

When Dad reached the middle stages of the disease and began wandering at night, we had to have caregivers with him 24 hours a day. Thankfully, dad's long-term care insurance covered it, but the costs quickly began depleting his policy. After a year or so, we decided to move him to assisted living at half the cost of 24-hour care in order to maintain a strong reserve in his policy. This was a very hard move, but it was the right move.

Moving your loved one to an independent care facility such as an assisted living facility can be a tough decision for all involved. You generally should take this step either when your loved one can no longer live alone or when your loved one's caregiver can no longer offer everything your loved one needs. The following checklist details some signs that you might want to consider moving your loved one to an independent living facility.

*Checklist: Signs an independent living facility could be beneficial*

**Your loved one:**

☐ Has started wandering often.

☐ Has become lost due to wandering.

☐ Has been brought home by police and/or neighbors because they were wandering and became disoriented.

☐ Has recently become more isolated, even depressed at times.

☐ Experiences little to no socialization during the day.

☐ Falls often.

☐ Becomes more and more confused on a daily basis.

☐ Has experienced difficulty cooking.

☐ Becomes violent (physically or verbally) or acts out frequently.

☐ Has started sundowning.

☐ Is not safe in their current living environment due to increasing symptoms of the disease; however, they can still perform basic activities of daily living independently or with minimal help.

**The caregiver:**

☐ Has begun losing sleep due to worrying about their loved one.

☐ Experiences extreme anger, sadness, and/or aggression because of stress and/or caregiver duties.

☐ Loses patience with their loved one often.

☐ Consistently gives up social or work events.

☐ Does not have time alone to rest and recuperate.

☐ Loses or gains weight due to stress.

☐ Experiences health problems.

☐ Has begun drinking alcohol, using drugs, or smoking to deal with stress.

☐ Can no longer keep up with their caregiver duties.

☐ Constantly worries their loved one will be injured due to escalating symptoms.

☐ Cannot physically help their loved one up if the individual falls.

☐ Has begun to resent their loved one for being ill.

The services that independent living facilities provide depend on the individual facility, and particularly on whether it specializes in memory care. However, the following checklist highlights some of the services these facilities frequently offer.

## Checklist: Services independent facilities often provide

☐ Housing (individual apartments, suites, or shared rooms)

☐ Housekeeping services

☐ Laundry services

☐ Three meals a day, often provided in a group setting; however, most facilities will allow residents to dine alone in their rooms if they want to

☐ Assistance with eating, such as if food needs to be cut into smaller pieces

☐ Twenty-four-hour staff for assistance with any needs that may arise

- ☐ Recreational activities and events

- ☐ Therapeutic activities, such as music therapy and pet therapy

- ☐ Activities to encourage exercise

- ☐ Relaxation activities such as yoga and meditation

- ☐ Help with bathing, dressing, and toileting as needed

- ☐ Assistance with medications, including reminding residents both when to take medications and what dose of medication to take

- ☐ Twenty-four-hour monitoring of the facility to prevent wandering

- ☐ Emergency call systems in all rooms

- ☐ Twenty-four-hour security around the facility

- ☐ Counseling and therapy services

- ☐ Physical and speech therapy

- ☐ Transportation to doctor's appointments

- ☐ Barber and beautician services for residents

- ☐ Limited health services

- ☐ Consultations from a nutritionist when needed

- ☐ Frequent visits from a nurse on staff to ensure the resident is doing well

Before choosing an independent facility, you and your loved one, if possible, should visit multiple times to get a feel for the atmosphere. You should also research the facility's services and individual policies. In addition, you may want to consider the following checklist of what to look for in an independent care facility.

*Checklist: Questions to consider when looking for an independent living facility*

- ☐ Do they have a special unit/facility for individuals with Alzheimer's disease?

- ☐ Do they accept residents in the early stages of Alzheimer's disease?

☐ What behaviors will result in a resident being asked to leave?

☐ Will residents who progress into a later stage of Alzheimer's disease need to move out, or does the facility have the ability to care for them?

☐ Do they offer hospice services if needed? Or will the person need to be transferred to a nursing home?

☐ What kind of training does the staff have in caring for residents with dementia/ Alzheimer's disease?

☐ Do they offer any activities specifically geared toward memory retention?

☐ Do residents have single apartments or will they share with others?

☐ How many residents are normally in a living area together?

☐ What is the ratio of staff to residents?

☐ How often do nurses check on residents?

☐ Do they accept residents in wheelchairs?

☐ Do they accept residents with oxygen tanks?

☐ Do common rooms, activity centers, offices, etc. all look the same, or do they have distinct design features to help eliminate confusion?

☐ Are there options for prepared food if residents do not want to cook?

☐ Are the grounds and rooms of the facility maintained well? Or are they run down and dirty?

☐ What are the outdoor areas of the facility like? Is the facility near a busy street? Are there paths for walking?

☐ Is there a gate or barrier of some sort around the facility to dissuade wandering?

☐ Is the staff friendly and receptive when you visit?

☐ Are the staff members outgoing?

☐ Do the other residents at the facility look happy?

☐ Can you visit your loved one at any time or are there visiting hours?

☐ Do they provide outings so that residents can visit local stores or attractions? If so, how often do these outings happen?

☐ What is the supervision like on the outings? If your loved one gets confused and wanders, will there be enough staff to notice your loved one is no longer with the group?

☐ Does the facility accept your loved one's insurance plan?

☐ What extra costs are included at the facility that are not generally covered by insurance? For example, some activities or programs may not be covered by insurance.

☐ Does the facility currently have any citations against it?

☐ Has the facility had any citations in the past? If so, how serious were the citations, and how long ago did they occur?

☐ What is the facility's policy regarding medication? Do they hand out medication daily to residents, or are residents expected to keep their own medication?

☐ What is the facility's policy in the case of a medical emergency?

☐ Does each apartment have an emergency response system to easily call for help?

☐ What is the staff coverage/assistance like on weekends and holidays?

Independent living facilities are generally reserved for those who do not need skilled medical care but may require assistance in their day-to-day activities. As such, these facilities are typically more appropriate when your loved one is in the earlier stages of Alzheimer's disease.

## Going Out

When your loved one is in an assisted care facility, you will often be responsible for them when they need or want to venture out. Most trips will be to familiar locations such as the doctor's office, grocery store, or church. However, if your loved one is capable, you may choose to make some trips simply for your loved one's enjoyment.

When my dad was in assisted living, I was able to take him out to lunch once a week. He seemed to really enjoy these ventures outside the facility, and he loved the food. I often brought my young son with me, and it was a chance for Dad to really be able to act as a grandpa. All went well for five or six months. Then one day, I took dad to a new place that I thought he would like. The meal was perfect, Dad was actually conversing coherently, and we had a wonderful conversation. I dropped Dad off at his room in the assisted living facility and left feeling grateful for the day we had. An hour later, I received a call from the facility. Dad had hit someone. This was the first fight Dad was ever in. Completely unprovoked, he started punching people.

Dad had to be sent to a psychiatric facility. In meeting with the geriatric psychiatrist, I was told that taking Dad out of his environment could be triggering these episodes. The psychiatrist followed him around for a day and didn't notice anything unusual. Dad went back to assisted living. He hit someone else and was sent back to the psychiatric facility. In my state, the patient who has three psychiatric stays at a hospital can be denied entrance by any nursing home. Dad was at two. As a result, I not only had to end our outings, but had to fast-track my plans for moving Dad into a full-time care facility.

As this story demonstrates, your ability to take your loved one out will change as the disease progresses, and it's hard to know how they will react. In addition to short excursions, some occasions may require your loved one to travel or leave home for an extended period of time. These situations require extra effort and preparation.

## Special Occasions

Your loved one may be invited to special occasions such as holiday parties, family gatherings, graduations, or birthday parties. These events will likely be in an unfamiliar, loud, and crowded location. All of these qualities can increase stress, agitation, and confusion for your loved one. Ways to help your loved one adapt to this new or changed environment are listed below.

### Checklist: Participating in special occasions

☐ Inform people coming to the party about changes in your loved one's condition so they don't get too emotional and upset your loved one. Ask guests not to discuss your loved one's disease or health with your loved one, because this may also upset them.

☐ Prepare a place where your loved one can go to escape the noise and stimulation. Your loved one may need to rest or just be alone for a few minutes to help decrease confusion, anxiety, and exhaustion.

- ☐ Be prepared for your loved one to think they are attending a special occasion in the past. Encourage your loved one to talk about the past event. Do not try to correct or reorient them, because this may cause more confusion and anxiety.

- ☐ If your loved one is unable to participate in the entire event, choose to attend the portion of the event that is most meaningful to them.

- ☐ If your loved one is unable to attend the event, consider bringing the event to them. For example, if your loved one cannot attend a wedding, a visit from the bride and groom may prove special to your loved one.

- ☐ If your loved one is still at home, consider having the celebration at your loved one's home with just a small group of people. Multiple smaller parties will be easier for your loved one than one large party. Plan the party for your loved one's best time of day.

- ☐ If visitors will be staying in your loved one's home, make sure they are aware of potential hazards such as leaving out medications or creating clutter that your loved one may trip over.

- ☐ If you will be hosting a large party that your loved one will attend, prepare your loved one ahead of time by discussing your plans. Use simple sentences, and remind them frequently.

- ☐ Involve your loved one in the planning and preparations. Even if they can't contribute like they once did, they will enjoy being involved and feeling needed.

- ☐ Stick to favorite traditions rather than trying to do everything. For example, if the family's favorite tradition is frosting sugar cookies together, then make only sugar cookies and not all the other Christmas treats you might normally have.

- ☐ Enlist help from others both in preparations and in caregiving during the event. Ask others to bring food for a potluck-style meal.

- ☐ Plan quiet activities such as looking through a photo album rather than loud, boisterous activities such as playing games.

- ☐ If decorating for a holiday, choose a few subtle decorations that will not alter your loved one's environment too much. Too many decorations may cause confusion because of changes to visual cues.

☐ Secure decorations so they do not fall or pose a tripping or fire hazard to your loved one. Be sure to monitor all flammable decorations at all times when your loved one is present.

## Traveling

Some occasions, such as weddings or vacations, may require your loved one to travel by car or airplane. This will be another stressful situation for your loved one, especially if they have not flown or gone on long trips frequently in the past. The noise level, unfamiliar concourses, confined seating, and strange physical sensations will add to your loved one's confusion and stress level. Good tips to prepare for traveling with your loved one are listed below.

### Checklist: Traveling tips

☐ Allow extra time for every step of the trip, from packing to arrival.

☐ Pack important documents such as medication information, travel itineraries, and contact information. Keep at least one copy with your loved one in case they wander and get lost.

☐ Pack activities, snacks, and water in a small bag for your loved one.

☐ If possible, travel to known locations that are close to home. Plan to be away from home for only a few days.

☐ Travel during your loved one's best time of day, and choose the travel option that will cause the least anxiety for your loved one.

☐ Avoid traveling on peak travel days. It is also better to travel in the off-season when hotels and major activities will be less crowded.

☐ Avoid scheduling flights with tight connections, and try to fly direct if possible.

☐ Never let your loved one travel unattended. It is not the job of the airline employees to make sure your loved one stays safe. Consider bringing someone along who can help with the caregiving duties.

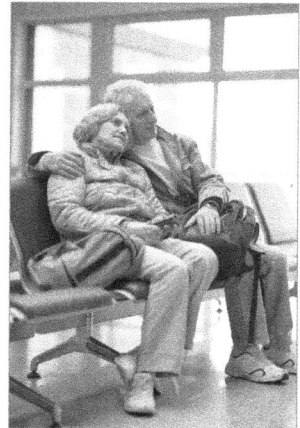

☐ Get a letter from the doctor stating that your loved one has a cognitive impairment. This will help ease tensions with airport security if your loved one has trouble following directions.

☐ Inform hotel and airline staff of your loved one's special needs before you arrive, and remind them of these needs when you arrive.

☐ Consider requesting wheelchair support at your gate so that you have an airport employee to accompany you. Special considerations such as this often require at least 48 hours' advance notice.

☐ Use the restroom before getting on the plane to avoid having to use the on-board lavatory. If you think your loved one will need to use the bathroom on the plane, schedule the bathroom trip about an hour before the end of the flight to avoid needing the bathroom when the seatbelt sign is turned on for landing.

☐ Preboard the aircraft, and choose a middle or window seat for your loved one and an aisle seat for yourself so your loved one cannot wander without you noticing. If possible, sit on a side with only two seats.

☐ Request a hotel room designed for people with disabilities. Share a room with your loved one, and sleep in the bed nearest the door. Consider bringing along a travel door alarm to warn you if your loved one tries to leave the room.

☐ When you arrive at your hotel room or other accommodations, assess the room or house for hazards and remove them. If you are staying at someone's home, kindly ask them if you can remove the hazards for the duration of your stay.

☐ Stick to your loved one's normal schedule as much as possible. Keep meal and bed times the same, and bring along a favorite pillow or pair of pajamas.

☐ If you are enrolled in an emergency response program such as MedicAlert® + Safe Return®, alert the program that you will be traveling. Keep a recent photo of your loved one with you to show to people if they get lost.

☐ Learn contact details for and directions to medical services at your destination.

☐ If your loved one is in an advanced stage of disease, suffers from incontinence, cannot perform most activities of daily living on their own, or gets confused easily, consider staying home.

# Moving to a Full-Time Care Facility

Full-time care facilities are generally either nursing homes or settings very similar to nursing homes that specialize in memory loss. If your loved one requires medical attention, 24-hour care, assistance with walking and dressing, and/or around-the-clock supervision, a full-time care facility could be helpful. These facilities employ teams of nurses, social workers, therapists, nutritionists, and doctors to aid residents in their day-to-day needs. In addition, most nursing homes have common areas where activities are held, as well as options for communal dining so that residents can socialize with one another if they so choose.

After Dad's aggressive episodes at the assisted living facility, I knew I had to decide which full-time care facility I wanted to place him in. Dad was already on waiting lists for the best nursing homes, but no spots were open. A nursing home with a "below average" rating was close to my home, so close that it was within walking distance. I talked to the geriatric psychiatrist and agonized over what to do. He told me, "Even if it was the Ritz Carlton, your dad would not know. You have to do what is best for you." I placed Dad in the nursing home, and I wasn't happy. However, I also recognized that I would not be happy with any facility. Dad was safe and fed and not in any visible emotional distress or pain. Sometimes that is the best we can do.

Like me, many individuals view full-time care facilities, such as nursing homes, as either unnecessary or negative in some way. Due to this misconception, many caregivers and family members feel extreme guilt when a loved one with Alzheimer's disease is placed in a long-term care facility. The truth, however, is that your loved one will likely need some form of full-time care toward the later stages of their disease. The checklist below highlights some signs that your loved one might benefit from a long-term care facility.

*Checklist: Signs your loved one could benefit from a long-term care facility*

**Your loved one:**

☐ Has begun wandering during the day and at night.

☐ Has been injured due to wandering.

☐ Needs daily medical assistance from a professional.

☐ Has a serious medical condition in addition to Alzheimer's disease.

- [ ] Needs 24-hour care and supervision.

- [ ] Has begun aspirating or choking on their food regularly.

- [ ] Is now bedridden.

- [ ] Is incontinent and/or is using objects other than the toilet for voiding.

- [ ] Is becoming sexually, physically, or emotionally abusive.

- [ ] Has lost the ability to communicate their needs (through speech, hand gestures, or writing).

- [ ] Needs frequent assistance walking or standing.

- [ ] Is no longer safe in their environment.

- [ ] Requires pain management, medical care, and/or hospice care.

- [ ] Has symptoms that are becoming too much for their caregiver to manage.

- [ ] Needs physical assistance with eating.

- [ ] Requires daily management of medications.

The services provided by long-term care facilities will vary based on the type of institution. For example, specialized units called memory care units will have services geared toward individuals with Alzheimer's disease, whereas nursing homes will generally have fewer services available that work specifically with memory loss. Some nursing homes, however, do have units that specialize in Alzheimer's care. The following checklist discusses some of the services provided by full-time care facilities.

### Checklist: Services provided at full-time care facilities

- [ ] Specialized medical care

- [ ] Twenty-four-hour-a-day nursing services

- [ ] Assistance taking medications

- [ ] Prescription of new medications

- [ ] Wound care

- ☐ Preventative care and access to necessary immunizations, such as flu and pneumonia vaccines

- ☐ Arrangements with local hospitals in case of a medical emergency

- ☐ Palliative care (some facilities will provide hospice services, but in many cases, you will need to arrange this yourself if they allow it)

- ☐ Dental care (some facilities will provide monthly access to a dentist, but this is not the case in all areas, so check with the individual facility)

- ☐ Health and nutrition management

- ☐ Three balanced meals a day (generally served in a dining room, but residents can request that food be served in their room)

- ☐ Help with any feeding needs

- ☐ Housekeeping

- ☐ Laundry services

- ☐ Assistance bathing and dressing

- ☐ Monitoring and assistance with personal hygiene

- ☐ Assistance with toileting and the use of garments for incontinence

- ☐ Recreational activities with other residents

- ☐ Activities and programs to promote physical exercise

- ☐ Memory retention activities

- ☐ Religious and cultural programs and activities

- ☐ Physical therapy and speech therapy

- ☐ A secure environment with 24-hour-a-day monitoring

- ☐ Management of behavior changes and outbursts

- ☐ Design features organized so as not to be visually distracting or confusing (e.g., all hallways and offices do not look the same)

☐ Large, descriptive signs labeling offices, bathrooms, dining rooms, and resident quarters to help in identification and the reduction of confusion

When deciding on a full-time care facility, you should visit the facility at different parts of the day and week to see how the staff interacts with residents, how activities such as meal times are conducted, and how the environment changes with different staff and activities. For example, visit the facility in the morning and at meal times to see how much the noise volume increases. You can also go on the Internet to check how the home is rated overall for service and quality. The following checklist highlights some areas to pay particular attention to when selecting a full-time care facility.

### Checklist: Questions to consider when looking for a full-time care facility

☐ Do they admit individuals with Alzheimer's disease?

☐ Do they have a special Alzheimer's disease unit? If so, how is it different than the other units?

☐ Can residents who progress to the later stages of Alzheimer's disease stay at the facility, or do they have to move?

☐ Is the staff trained to work with patients with Alzheimer's disease?

☐ Will the facility provide you with a sample care plan for a resident who has Alzheimer's disease?

☐ Do they provide any activities aimed at residents with memory loss?

☐ Does the facility perform background checks on all employees? What are their hiring restrictions in light of these background checks? In other words, if a person has ever been suspected of abuse or mistreatment, will the facility still hire them?

☐ What is the facility's policy for staff members who use physical force against a resident? (It should be zero-tolerance.)

☐ What kind of security is in place if a resident wanders or becomes confused?

☐ Where are the cameras at the facility located? Will you be able to have access to the footage if needed (such as in cases of suspected abuse)?

- ☐ Does the facility have activities available every day?

- ☐ How much social interaction do residents have with staff and with one another?

- ☐ Do residents share rooms with one another, or are single rooms available?

- ☐ Is there an outside area for residents?

- ☐ How are meal times handled?

- ☐ How many people are available to help residents eat? (Patients cannot use silverware at some stages of the disease.)

- ☐ Can residents eat in their rooms if they wish?

- ☐ How does the staff promote and/or monitor healthy nutrition?

- ☐ What forms of nutritional assessment will be conducted? How often will these assessments be conducted?

- ☐ Are families encouraged to participate in activities, meal times, and overall care?

- ☐ How are medications stored? (They should be locked and kept far away from residents.)

- ☐ Do the residents at the facility appear to be happy?

- ☐ Are the current residents well-groomed and dressed appropriately?

- ☐ Is the staff friendly and respectful?

- ☐ Is the setup/design of the facility easy to navigate?

- ☐ What are the visiting hours? Do those hours work with your schedule?

- ☐ What is the ratio of nurses and doctors to residents?

- ☐ What is the ratio of social workers to residents?

- ☐ What is the ratio of nurses (RNs) to staff/CNAs to staff on weekdays and on the weekends?

- ☐ What is the employee turnover rate?

- ☐ What policies are in place in case of medical emergency?

☐ Does the facility provide hospice services if they are needed?

☐ Can your loved one's living space be decorated in any way they choose?

☐ What religious and/or cultural services are in place for residents?

☐ What doctors will be caring for your loved one, and will you be able to meet and approve them before any care is given?

☐ What is the reputation of the facility?

☐ Does the facility currently have any citations pending against it? If so, how serious are the citations?

☐ Has the facility had citations in the past?

☐ Is the facility covered by your loved one's insurance provider?

☐ How long is the waiting list to get a bed at the facility? Will it be longer if your loved one is on Medicaid?

☐ How will you be billed for services? What extras should you expect on top of the monthly fee (i.e., haircuts, activities, incontinence briefs, gloves)?

☐ Can you speak to current staff, residents, and family members of residents before you choose the facility?

☐ How is the facility designed? Do all the hallways and common areas look the same, or are there distinguishing features to prevent confusion?

☐ Is the facility overly noisy? What is the facility's policy on noise control?

☐ What types of activities are offered to residents? How frequently are they held?

## Memory Care Units

Some assisted living and long-term care facilities are specifically tailored to residents with Alzheimer's disease and are called memory care units, special care units, or memory support programs. These units are generally set apart from the other areas of the facility and have dedicated staff. Short-term or long-term care facilities that offer specialized programs for individuals with Alzheimer's disease can be very beneficial for your loved one. Your loved one will be around others who have memory difficulties, and the staff will be trained to work with individuals who have dementia.

If you are unsure whether a facility you are considering has a program for residents with Alzheimer's disease, you can always check their website to see if they have information there, or you can call the facility and ask. The following checklist details some of the features of memory care units.

## Checklist: Features of memory care units

☐ All residents have either dementia or Alzheimer's disease.

☐ Staff has specialized training to care for individuals with dementia or Alzheimer's disease.

☐ Staff receives frequent training in order to stay knowledgeable about new research, findings, and changes to suggested care practices.

☐ Activities and games are aimed at memory retention.

☐ Enhanced safety protocols are in place.

☐ Large signs and other measures are in place to help decrease disorientation and confusion.

☐ Unit often provides a higher degree of individualized attention.

☐ Unit features private or semi-private living areas.

☐ Rooms are designed to promote resident independence.

☐ Both nurses and social workers provide 24-hour supervision and care.

☐ The ratio of nurses and doctors to residents to provide specialized and dedicated care is high.

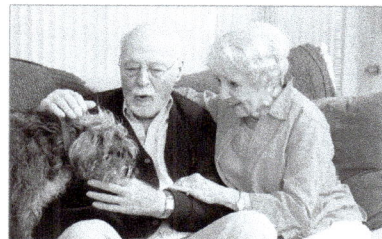

☐ More pet, music, art, and relaxation therapies are available.

☐ Personalized programs are tailored to help individual residents.

☐ A larger emphasis is placed on recreational and social activities to promote stimulation and avoid sedentary activities.

As previously mentioned, memory care units are designed specifically for individuals with Alzheimer's disease or other forms of dementia. Given this characteristic, a facility like this would be an ideal place for your loved one to live if you can find one in your area that is covered by your loved one's insurance or is otherwise affordable.

## Psychiatric Facilities

If your loved one develops problems with aggression or violence, they may be placed in a psychiatric facility, especially if they were in an assisted living or long-term care facility and injured a caregiver or another resident. Care facilities must protect their workers and residents, and having a resident who is a danger to others is a liability many facilities will not tolerate. If you are unable to handle your loved one's care outside of a long-term care facility, your loved one may be placed in a psychiatric facility and held involuntarily until the situation subsides. To understand more about psychiatric facilities, see the checklists below.

*Checklist: Reasons your loved one may be placed in a psychiatric facility*

- ☐ Biting

- ☐ Hitting

- ☐ Pushing

- ☐ Cursing/swearing

- ☐ Pulling hair

- ☐ Delusions

- ☐ Paranoia

- ☐ Hallucinations

- ☐ Fighting

- ☐ Threatening someone with a sharp object

- ☐ Spitting

- ☐ Mood swings

- ☐ Threatening to commit suicide

☐ Yelling

☐ Stomping on someone

## Checklist: What to expect from a psychiatric facility

☐ Your loved one may be held for 72 hours or more without your approval.

☐ Your loved one should be assessed by a physician.

☐ The physician will likely try different combinations of medications to control aggressive or psychiatric symptoms.

☐ The physician will likely try to identify triggers for psychiatric or aggressive behavior. For individuals with Alzheimer's disease, seemingly unlikely triggers can cause aggression, such as a change in environment, asking your loved one to change clothing, or trying to force them to take medication or take a bath.

☐ Your loved one may be placed in a solitary room.

☐ Your loved one may be restrained by the arms and/or legs.

☐ Your loved one's health and mental acuity may decline rapidly after a stay in a psychiatric facility, or it may improve if the staff finds a better drug regimen.

☐ Your loved one may require a court order to be released from the facility.

☐ Your loved one will likely have a harder time finding another long-term care facility to take them after their release from the psychiatric facility.

Many individuals with Alzheimer's disease suffer through a period of aggression. Therefore, you and your family may want to be prepared for this by choosing a psychiatric facility that you would like your loved one transported to in case of emergency. Once you have made this choice, notify your loved one's assisted living or long-term care facility of your decision and ask them to honor your wishes should your loved one need to be placed in a psychiatric facility. Questions to ask when choosing a psychiatric facility are listed below.

## Checklist: Questions to ask when choosing a psychiatric facility

☐ What is the physician-to-patient ratio? What is the nurse-to-patient ratio?

☐ Are physicians available for consultations and appointments over the weekend and on holidays? Or will your loved one be required to wait over the weekend or holiday before being assessed?

☐ Do the physicians, nurses, and other employees have experience dealing with behaviors of individuals with advanced Alzheimer's disease?

☐ Do the physicians have experience successfully finding medication combinations that can control behavioral changes in your loved one without making them lethargic?

☐ Does the facility have a standard protocol for dealing with acts of aggression? If so, what is it? Is it something you are comfortable with?

☐ What is the facility's policy on solitary confinement?

☐ What is the facility's policy on restraints?

☐ Does the facility have a history of reported abuse?

☐ Are there adequate opportunities for mental stimulation and physical activity?

☐ Will the facility help your loved one with activities of daily living (e.g., bathing, eating, toileting) if your loved one is unable to do them on their own?

☐ Will you be allowed to visit your loved one in the psychiatric facility? If so, what are the visiting hours?

☐ What is the overall environment of the psychiatric facility? Does it provide a calm atmosphere? Are residents too isolated?

☐ What fees are associated with a voluntary stay versus an involuntary stay at the psychiatric facility?

☐ Will the facility accept your loved one's healthcare or long-term care insurance?

☐ How close is the psychiatric facility to your house and your loved one's care facility?

☐ What is the facility's policy about releasing your loved one into your care if they were placed in the psychiatric facility by an assisted living or long-term care facility?

Although having your loved one committed to a psychiatric facility is difficult emotionally, knowing what to expect and being prepared for this possibility will make the transition easier for you. Having a plan in place that your family, your loved one, and your loved one's care facility agree on will make the transition much smoother, and it will prevent any surprises that would cause undue emotional stress.

# Elder Abuse

No matter what your loved one's living arrangements are, it is important to be aware of the possibility for elder abuse. Individuals with Alzheimer's disease are often frustrating to work with because they do not understand, are forgetful, and may be prone to violence or defiance. These characteristics may cause caregivers to abuse the individual with Alzheimer's disease in order to get them to cooperate. Individuals with Alzheimer's disease are extremely susceptible to elder abuse because they often don't recognize that they are being abused, do not have the verbal or cognitive skills to report the abuse, and think that no one will believe their report of abuse because of their frequent confusion.

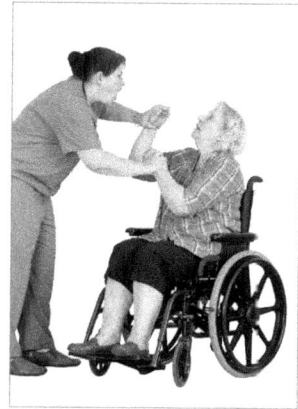

Elder abuse can come in many different forms, as listed below, and it can occur as a single act or repeated acts. In most cases of repeated abuse, the abuser is someone the individual knows well, such as a close family member or friend. Elder abuse is also common in long-term care facilities, because caregivers often do not have the time or resources to handle the complex behaviors associated with Alzheimer's disease.

## Checklist: Types of elder abuse

☐ **Physical abuse:** Physical injury because of beating, lashing, cutting, burning, or other physical assault.

☐ **Emotional abuse:** Emotional disturbance because of shouting, verbal insults, threats, harassment, or intimidation.

☐ **Sexual abuse:** Inappropriate touching that is forced on the individual or that they cannot consent to or understand; this can also include inappropriate sexual comments.

☐ **Financial abuse:** Withholding finances that will provide essential care for the individual, or using the individual's finances in a way that is a disadvantage to the individual but an advantage to someone else. (Such abuse is often a result of inappropriate use of a power of attorney or of strangers scamming an unsuspecting older adult with dementia.)

☐ **Neglect:** Intentionally or unintentionally withholding food, water, shelter, medical care, hygiene care, and other basic necessities; this increases the individual's risk of physical or emotional harm.

☐ **Confinement:** Restraining or isolating the individual against their wishes.

☐ **Medical abuse:** Inappropriate prescription or withholding of antipsychotics and other prescription medications, restraints, catheters, and/or similar medical treatments.

Your loved one may be at risk for abuse both at home and at a care center. Caregivers, family members, and friends may abuse your loved one out of ignorance, frustration, or selfishness. How can you recognize if your loved one is being abused? You can look for some of the signs listed below.

## Checklist: Signs of abuse

☐ Noticeable injuries such as bruises, broken bones, abrasions, or burns

☐ Matching bruises on the arms or throat (may indicate rough grabbing)

☐ Small round burn marks (may indicate being touched with a burning cigarette)

☐ Unexplained pain when moving

☐ Unexplained withdrawal from social activities

☐ Sudden changes in alertness or depression symptoms

☐ Bruises around the breast or genital areas

☐ Unexpected or unexplained withdrawals from a checking or savings account

☐ Increased occurrence of unpaid bills

☐ A new friend asks to help with your loved one's banking

- [ ] Sudden changes to legal documents such as power of attorney or will

- [ ] Pressure ulcers

- [ ] Poor hygiene

- [ ] Unexpected weight loss

- [ ] Frequent arguments between your loved one and a specific person

Detecting abuse of an individual with Alzheimer's disease may be especially difficult because some of the signs of abuse, such as withdrawal or depression, are also common with disease progression even in the absence of abuse. Your consistent involvement in your loved one's life will allow you to more readily differentiate signs of abuse from signs of disease progression. As a caregiver and someone concerned about your loved one's physical and emotional safety, there are several ways you can help prevent or stop abuse, as stated in the checklist below.

### Checklist: Ways to prevent elder abuse

- [ ] Be involved in your loved one's life.

- [ ] Undergo training in how to deal with the challenging behaviors that accompany Alzheimer's disease.

- [ ] Be aware of the care your loved one is receiving and the people your loved one interacts with daily; perform background or reference checks for people who will be caring for your loved one.

- [ ] Don't be afraid to ask questions of other caregivers and family members if you notice new injuries or behaviors.

- [ ] Ensure that your loved one's finances are being used for their best interests and not the interests of others.

- [ ] Be aware of individuals asking for money, including "salesmen" and other scammers. These individuals may use force or threats to con money out of your loved one.

- [ ] If you notice a caregiver that seems burned out or overburdened, offer to give them a break or refer them to a support group.

☐ If you suspect that your loved one is being abused, call national or state adult protective services or the police department. They will investigate your suspicions and bring charges against guilty parties if needed.

Keep in mind that because of your loved one's mental decline, you as a caregiver may also be susceptible to abuse by your loved one. Individuals with Alzheimer's disease may become aggressive and lash out at caregivers without provocation. No individual should have to live with the threat of abuse, even if it is coming from a loved one with dementia. If your loved one becomes abusive to you or other family members, seek help from medical professionals and loved ones.

# Conclusion

Many options exist for living arrangements for your loved one with Alzheimer's disease, and each comes with its own set of concerns related to the independence and safety of your loved one. Your loved one can usually stay home in the early stages of the disease, but as things progress, they will likely need to move in with a caregiver or move to an assisted living or long-term care facility. These decisions are not easy to make, and they can prove stressful to you as a caregiver. Discussing options with your loved one while they are still mentally able to make decisions may help. In addition, knowing what questions to ask and what features to look for in care facilities can make the process more navigable. There are numerous resources that can help you organize care for your loved one, so you do not have to go through the process alone.

Ultimately, Alzheimer's disease affects not only the individual who has the disease, but the family and friends of that individual as well. The decisions you must make are difficult, but they are necessary to protect your loved one and give those who care about them of mind.

# ABOUT THE AUTHORS

## Laura Town

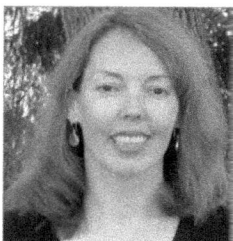

Laura Town has authored numerous publications of special interest to the aging population. She has expertise in the field of finance as a co-author on *Finance: Foundations of Financial Institutions and Management* published by John Wiley and Sons, and she has contributed to several online nursing courses and texts. She has also written for the American Medical Writers Association, and her work has been published by the American Society of Journalists and Authors. As an editor, Laura has worked with Pearson Education, Prentice Hall, McGraw-Hill Higher Education, John Wiley and Sons, and the University of Pennsylvania to create both on-ground and online courses and texts. She is currently the President-Elect of the Indiana chapter of the American Medical Writers Association.

## Karen Kassel

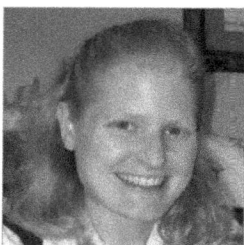

Karen Kassel received her Ph.D. in pharmacology from the Department of Pharmacology and Experimental Neurosciences at the University of Nebraska Medical Center in Omaha, where she was the recipient of an American Heart Association fellowship and several regional and national awards for her research on G protein-coupled receptor signaling in airways. She then pursued post-doctoral research projects at the University of North Carolina–Chapel Hill and the University of Kansas Medical Center, again receiving fellowships from the PhRMA Foundation and the American Heart Association, respectively. She has published research in the *American Journal of Pathology, Journal of Biological Chemistry*, and *Journal of Pharmacology and Experimental Therapeutics*. In 2012, Karen joined the editorial staff at WilliamsTown Communications, an editing firm that specializes in educational products for undergraduate- and graduate-level students. At WTC, Karen specializes in producing educational products related to the sciences and healthcare. In addition, Karen recently became board-certified for editing life sciences (BELS-certified).

## Amanda Boyle

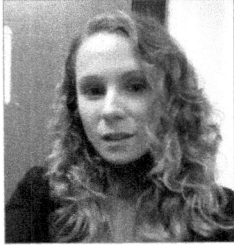

Amanda Boyle earned her master's degree in English from the State University of New York at New Paltz. During her time there, she presented academic essays at numerous literary conferences in the United States and Europe. Amanda has been a writer and editor for WilliamsTown Communications since 2011. She has overseen the production of online courses for various disciplines, including psychology and nursing, and has served as a writer in both subject areas. As an editor, Amanda has worked on management, business, science, and nursing textbooks.

# A NOTE FROM THE AUTHORS

Thank you for purchasing our book! Worldwide, over 40 million people suffer from Alzheimer's disease, and that number is expected to increase significantly within the next 15 years. In the United States, five million people have the disease, and that is expected to triple by the year 2050.

Despite these large numbers, you may feel alone. I (Laura) know that when I started caring for my father, who had early-onset Alzheimer's disease, I felt alone. Although my father has passed away, I am haunted by what he suffered and how difficult it was to care for him. However, now I know that there are people, resources, and organizations that can help others going through this same struggle.

We recognize that caregivers have emotional, physical, and financial challenges. We hope that the information in the *Alzheimer's Roadmap* series will ease some of your stress. The steps included in this book can help you recognize the signs that a new living situation is needed, as well as aid you in assessing that living situation for safety and quality. All of the steps may not apply to every situation, but they will stimulate your thinking and get you progressing forward in the moving process. In addition, we have included resources at the end of each book to provide additional information to help you through this process.

If you have any questions for us, feel free to post them on Laura Town's Amazon Author Central page or reach out via Twitter: @laurawtown, @KarenKassel1, and @AmandaLBoyle. We would appreciate it if you would take the time to review our book on Amazon, as our book's visibility on Amazon depends on reviews.

## More Titles from Laura Town and Karen Kassel

☐ *Long-Term Care Insurance, Power of Attorney, Wealth Management, and Other First Steps*

☐ *Advance Directives, Durable Power of Attorney, Wills, and Other Legal Considerations*

☐ *Dementia, Alzheimer's Disease Stages, Treatment Options, and Other Medical Considerations*

☐ *Home Safety Checklist Guide and Caregiver Resources for Medication Safety, Driving, and Wandering* (contains some information also included in this book)

- [ ] *Home Care, Long-Term Care, Memory Care Units, and Other Living Arrangements* (contains some information also included in this book)

- [ ] *Caregiver Resources for Helping with Activities of Daily Living*

- [ ] *Nutrition for Brain Health: Fighting Dementia*

# RESOURCES

## Information Regarding Care Options

**Alzheimer's Association Information on Home Services**
Phone: 800-272-3900
Website: http://www.alz.org/care/

**Alzheimer's Association Information on Caregiver Support Groups**
Website: http://www.alz.org/care/alzheimers-dementia-support-groups.asp

**Caring Bridge**
Website: http://www.caringbridge.org/
*Helps you coordinate caregiving tasks with family and friends

**Eldercare Locator**
Website: http://www.eldercare.gov/Eldercare.NET/Public/Index.aspx
*Helps locate long- and short-term care facilities in your area

**National Care Planning Council**
Website: http://www.longtermcarelink.net/a7nursinghome.htm
*Provides links to care providers, services, and advisors broken down by state

**Nursing Home Compare**
Website: http://www.medicare.gov/nursinghomecompare/search.html
*Provides information about every nursing home in the U.S. that is Medicare or Medicaid certified

**Senior Living**
Website: http://www.seniorliving.org/lifestyles/memory-care/
*Provides a list of long-term, short-term, and memory care facilities in your area, as well as resources for local homecare services

**Meals on Wheels America**
413 N. Lee Street
Alexandria, VA 22314
Phone: 888-998-6325
Fax: 703-548-5274
Email: info@mealsonwheelsamerica.org
Website: www.mealsonwheelsamerica.org
*Allows you to search for your local Meals on Wheels program

# Caregiver Agreement Examples

## Utah
http://www.caregivers.utah.gov/sample_contract.htm

## North Carolina
http://elder-clinic.law.wfu.edu/files/2010/11/CareAgreement.pdf

## Maine
http://www.maine.gov/dhhs/ofi/documents/LTC-Personal-Support-Agreement.pdf

# Information about Emergency Alert Systems

## Philips Lifeline
Phone: 855-214-1363
Website: www.lifelinesys.com

## Medic Alert + Alzheimer's Association Safe Return
2323 Colorado Boulevard
Turlock, CA 95380
Phone: 888-572-8566
Fax: 800-863-3429
Website: www.medicalert.org/safereturn

## Silver Alert
The Alzheimer's Foundation of America has a list of programs by state here: http://www.alzfdn.org/EducationandCare/silver_alert.html.

Each state has its own program, so you will need to look up your state's information based on this list.

## Other emergency alert companies:
- Alert1
- Bay Alarm Medical
- Care Innovations Link
- Life Alert
- LifeFone
- LifeStation
- Medical Guardian
- MobileHelp
- Rescue Alert

To see a comparison of these companies, visit http://medical-alert-systems-review.toptenreviews.com/.

# General Information about Alzheimer's Disease

### Alzheimer's Association

225 N. Michigan Avenue, Floor 17
Chicago, IL 60601-7633
Phone: 800-272-3900
Fax: 866-699-1246
Email: info@alz.org
Website: http://www.alz.org

### Alzheimer's Foundation of America

322 Eighth Avenue, 7th Floor
New York, NY 10001
Phone: 866-232-8484
Fax: 646-638-1546
Website: www.alzfdn.org

## Other

### American Association of Poison Control Centers

515 Kind Street, Suite 510
Alexandria, VA 22314
Phone: 800-222-1222
Email: info@aapcc.org
Website: http://www.aapcc.org
*Allows you to search for your local poison control center

### Other books in the Alzheimer's Roadmap series

- *Long-Term Care Insurance, Power of Attorney, Wealth Management, and Other First Steps*

- *Advance Directives, Durable Power of Attorney, Wills, and Other Legal Considerations*

- *Dementia, Alzheimer's Disease Stages, Treatment Options, and Other Medical Considerations*

- *Home Safety Checklist Guide and Caregiver Resources for Medication Safety, Driving, and Wandering* (contains some information also included in this book)

- *Home Care, Long-Term Care, Memory Care Units, and Other Living Arrangements* (contains some information also included in this book)

- *Caregiver Resources for Helping with Activities of Daily Living*

- *Nutrition for Brain Health: Fighting Dementia*

# REFERENCE LIST

Administration on Aging. (2013). Home health care. Retrieved from http://www.eldercare.gov/eldercare.net/public/resources/factsheets/home_health_care.aspx

Alzheimer's Association. (2012). Staying safe: Steps to take for a person with dementia. Retrieved from https://www.alz.org/national/documents/brochure_stayingsafe.pdf

Alzheimer's Compendium. (n.d.) Traveling with an Alzheimer's patient. Retrieved from http://www.alzcompend.info/?p=133

Alzheimer's Foundation of America. (2014). Excellence in design: Optimal living space for people with Alzheimer's disease and related dementias. Retrieved from http://www.alzfdn.org/documents/ExcellenceinDesign_Report.pdf

Alzheimer's Hope. (2014). Wandering. Retrieved from http://www.alzheimershope.com/symptoms_strategies/wandering.php

Alzheimer's Society (2013). Mistreatment and abuse of people with dementia. Retrieved from http://www.alzheimers.org.uk/site/scripts/documents_info.php?documentID=422

Alzheimer Society Canada. (2014). Holidays and special occasions. Retrieved from http://www.alzheimer.ca/en/Living-with-dementia/Staying-connected/Holidays-and-special-occasions

Alzheimer Society of Manitoba. (2006). Fact sheet: Special occasions. Retrieved from http://www.alzheimer.mb.ca/wp-content/uploads/2013/09/Special-Occasions.pdf

American Academy of Orthopaedic Surgeons. (2012). Guidelines for preventing falls. Retrieved from http://orthoinfo.aaos.org/topic.cfm?topic=A00135

American Association of Retired Persons (AARP). (2011). 6 signs of caregiver burnout. Retrieved from http://www.aarp.org/relationships/caregiving-resource-center/info-12-2011/caregiver-burnout.1.html

Assisted Living Federation of America. (2013). Assisted living community evaluation checklist. Retrieved from http://www.alfa.org/alfa/Checklist_for_Evaluating_Communities.asp

Barak, Y., & Aizenberg, D. (2002). Suicide amongst Alzheimer's disease patients: A 10-year survey. *Dementia and Geriatric Cognitive Disorders, 14*(2), 101–103.

Care Pathways. (2014). Home care agency checklist. Retrieved from
    http://www.carepathways.com/checklist-hc.cfm

Centers for Medicare & Medicaid Services. (2013). Your guide to choosing a nursing
    home or other long-term care. Retrieved from http://www.medicare.gov/
    Pubs/pdf/02174.pdf

Family Caregiver Alliance. (2012). Personal care agreements: How to compensate a
    family member for providing care. Retrieved from https://caregiver.org/
    personal-care-agreements

Fisher Center for Alzheimer's Research Foundation. (2014). Assisted living facilities.
    Retrieved from http://www.alzinfo.org/08/treatment-care/assisted-living-
    facilities

Fodrini-Johnson, L. (n.d.). Family caregiver agreements: When a family member is
    paid. Retrieved from http://www.caremanager.org/why-care-management/
    consumer-librarylinksvideos/family-caregiver-agreements-when-a-family-
    member-is-paid/

Gross, J. (2008, October 6). Why hire a geriatric care manager? *New York Times*.
    Retrieved from http://newoldage.blogs.nytimes.com/2008/10/06/why-hire-a-
    geriatric-care-manager/?_php=true&_type=blogs&_php=true&_type=blogs&_
    php=true&_type=blogs&_php=true&_type=blogs&_r=3&

Heerema, E. (2013). Elder abuse and Alzheimer's disease: Types, indicators,
    prevention and response to elder abuse. *About Health*. Retrieved from
    http://alzheimers.about.com/od/legalissues/a/Elder-Abuse-And-Alzheimers-
    Disease.htm

————. (2014). What to do when someone with dementia talks about suicide.
    *About Health*. Retrieved from http://alzheimers.about.com/od/
    behaviormanagement/a/What-To-Do-When-Someone-With-Dementia-Talks-
    About-Suicide.htm

Mayo Clinic. (2013). Alzheimer's: When to stop driving. Retrieved from
    http://www.mayoclinic.org/healthy-living/caregivers/in-depth/alzheimers/art-
    20044924?pg=1

National Association of Professional Geriatric Care Managers. (2014). What you
    need to know. Retrieved from http://www.caremanager.org/why-care-
    management/what-you-should-know/

National Institute on Aging. (2010). Home safety for people with Alzheimer's
    disease. Retrieved from http://www.nia.nih.gov/sites/default/files/home_
    safety_for_people_with_alzheimers_disease_2.pdf

———. (2011). Driving and dementia: Health professionals can play an important role. Retrieved from http://www.nia.nih.gov/alzheimers/features/driving-and-dementia-health-professionals-can-play-important-role

———. (2012). Caring for a person with Alzheimer's disease. Retrieved from http://www.nia.nih.gov/sites/default/files/caring_for_a_person_with_alzheimers_disease_0.pdf

National Institutes of Health. (2012). Alzheimer's caregiving: What to do every day. Retrieved from http://nihseniorhealth.gov/alzheimerscare/dailyactivities/01.html

Seyfried, L. S., Kales, H. C., Ignacio, R. V., Conwell, Y., & Valenstein, M. (2011). Predictors of suicide in patients with dementia. *Alzheimer's & Dementia*, 7(6), 567–573.

"Staying safe: Wandering and the Alzheimer's patient." (2012). *Dementia Today*. Retrieved from http://www.dementiatoday.com/staying-safe-wandering-and-the-alzheimers-patient/

The Hartford Financial Services Group. (2010). At the crossroads: Family conversations about Alzheimer's disease, dementia and driving. Retrieved from http://hartfordauto.thehartford.com/UI/Downloads/Crossroads.pdf

———. (2010). The calm before the storm: Family conversations about disaster planning, caregiving, Alzheimer's disease, and dementia. Retrieved from http://hartfordauto.thehartford.com/UI/Downloads/CalmBeforeStorm Bro.pdf

www.ingramcontent.com/pod-product-compliance
Lightning Source LLC
Chambersburg PA
CBHW081649270326
41933CB00018B/3409